The Canine Herbal Remedies Bible

The Complete Guide to Holistic Canine Herbalism
with Clinically Proven & Effective Protocols
for Common Canine Conditions
to Protect Your Dog's Health & Longevity

LINCOLN FLEMING

Table of Contents

Disclaimer

This book is intended for informational purposes only and should not be used as a substitute for professional veterinary advice. Always consult with a veterinarian, especially one specializing in herbal medicine, to receive guidance tailored to your dog's health and well-being. The use of herbs carries risks and potential side effects, and a qualified professional can better advise you on safe and effective options for your pet.

Introduction

If you're reading this, chances are you're passionate about your dog's well-being. You want the best for your furry companion, and you're open to exploring alternative ways to care for them. In a world filled with medications and quick fixes, natural remedies are becoming an increasingly attractive option for pet owners who seek gentler, more holistic care. But, as you dive into the world of natural remedies for dogs, you might wonder: where do I start? How can herbs, which have been used for centuries, fit into my pet's modern health routine? The good news is that you're not alone, and you're in the right place.

This guide is designed to empower you. It's not just about replacing conventional medicine with herbs but understanding how the two can work together to support your dog's health in the most effective way. Whether your dog is suffering from anxiety, joint pain, skin issues, or digestive problems, natural remedies can offer solutions that work with their body's own healing mechanisms. You're about to embark on a journey that will give you the tools, knowledge, and confidence to make informed decisions about your pet's health. And don't worry—even if you're new to this approach, this guide will walk you through every step.

Before we dive into the world of herbs and their benefits, it's important to understand why natural remedies have become such a powerful trend in canine care. Let's start by exploring that.

WHY NATURAL REMEDIES FOR DOGS?

You might be wondering, "Why should I consider using natural remedies for my dog?" The answer lies in the growing awareness of how our pets' health is connected to the same principles that guide our own well-being. Natural remedies have been used for centuries across different cultures to address various health issues—humans and animals alike. Today, as pet owners, we're rediscovering the power of nature and looking beyond synthetic medications to provide our dogs with safer, gentler alternatives.

The Benefits of Using Herbs

Herbs offer a range of health benefits that can address both chronic and acute conditions in dogs. One of the biggest advantages is that they support the body's natural healing processes. Unlike pharmaceuticals, which often mask symptoms, herbs work to restore balance. For instance, chamomile can help act as a sedative and soothe anxiety and digestive issues, while turmeric is known for its anti-inflammatory properties, making it an excellent remedy for joint pain.

A study by the American Holistic Veterinary Medical Association found that many pet owners who incorporated herbal treatments alongside conventional care saw improvements in their pet's overall health, particularly with chronic issues like arthritis and skin allergies. Not only can herbs be gentler on your dog's system, but they can also prevent long-term reliance on medications that may have side effects.

When you choose herbal remedies, you're also embracing a more personalized approach to your dog's health. You can tailor treatments based on your pet's specific needs, creating a customized plan that supports them through all life stages. For instance, an older dog might benefit from a combination of turmeric for arthritis and milk thistle for liver support, while a younger, anxious dog might need calming herbs like valerian root or passionflower.

Understanding Holistic Care for Pets

Holistic care is about treating your dog as a whole—mind, body, and spirit. Instead of focusing on just the symptoms of an illness, it looks at the root causes and aims to improve overall well-being. This approach doesn't mean abandoning traditional veterinary care. On the contrary, holistic care complements conventional treatments, providing a balanced approach that can often lead to more effective results.

A key component of holistic pet care is prevention. Herbs can play a significant role in maintaining your dog's health, from boosting immunity to supporting digestion and reducing stress. By incorporating natural remedies into your dog's daily routine, you can prevent many issues before they escalate into more serious conditions.

How to Use This Guide Effectively

This guide is designed to be both educational and practical. You'll find it divided into sections that first explain the theory behind herbal medicine for dogs, followed by practical applications, including an encyclopedia of herbs and recipes you can easily prepare at home.

As you read through, start by understanding the foundational principles of herbal care. This will give you the knowledge to make informed decisions about what's best for your dog. Then, dive into the practical sections where you can learn about specific herbs and how to use them. By the end of this book, you'll feel confident in creating your own herbal remedies and knowing when to seek professional advice. Whether you're a seasoned pet owner or new to natural remedies, this guide will meet you where you are.

A BRIEF HISTORY OF HERBAL MEDICINE FOR ANIMALS

To fully appreciate the power of natural remedies for dogs, it helps to look at the history of herbal medicine for animals. The use of herbs for healing is not a new trend—it's deeply rooted in ancient traditions and has been used for thousands of years across different cultures.

Herbal Traditions in Canine Care

Herbal medicine dates back to the time when humans first domesticated animals. Early civilizations, from the Egyptians to the Chinese, used plants not only for their own healing but for their animals as well. For example, the ancient Egyptians were known to use herbs like garlic and aloe to treat their dogs' wounds and infections. In Traditional Chinese Medicine (TCM), herbs such as astragalus and ginseng were used to boost immunity and strengthen the body's vital energy, or "qi."

These ancient practices weren't based on guesswork. They were developed through careful observation of nature and how animals instinctively used certain plants to heal themselves. Dogs, like many animals, are naturally inclined to self-medicate. You've probably seen your dog chewing on grass when they feel unwell—that's their way of using nature to aid digestion or clear toxins. These natural instincts are the foundation of herbal medicine for animals.

Modern Developments in Holistic Veterinary Medicine

In recent decades, holistic veterinary medicine has gained credibility as more research supports the efficacy of herbal treatments. Veterinarians who specialize in holistic care often combine their traditional medical training with alternative therapies, offering a well-rounded approach to treating pets. Herbal remedies are now being used to manage everything from anxiety and arthritis to cancer, often with fewer side effects than conventional drugs.

Dr. Richard Pitcairn, a pioneer in holistic veterinary care, emphasizes the importance of integrating herbs into an overall wellness plan. In his book Dr. Pitcairn's Complete Guide to Natural Health for Dogs & Cats, he outlines how herbs can be used not only to treat illness but to prevent it by strengthening the body's natural defenses.

Today, holistic veterinarians and pet owners alike are discovering that natural remedies are a valuable tool in the fight against common canine ailments. From calming a nervous dog with lavender oil to easing arthritis with glucosamine and turmeric, herbs are playing an essential role in modern pet care.

The Science Behind Herbal Remedies

You might be wondering, "How exactly do herbs work in my dog's body?" The answer lies in the phytochemicals—natural compounds found in plants—that have specific effects on the body. These compounds can interact with your dog's immune system, reduce inflammation, and even act as antioxidants to protect against cell damage.

Research has shown that herbs like echinacea can stimulate the immune system, while milk thistle is well-known for its liver-protective properties. The science behind these remedies is growing, with many studies confirming the therapeutic effects of herbs for both humans and animals. For example, a study published in Veterinary Research Communications found that dogs treated with a combination of herbal supplements for joint pain showed significant improvement in mobility and reduced reliance on pain medications.

By incorporating herbal remedies into your dog's health routine, you're not just treating symptoms—you're addressing the root cause of the problem. Whether it's boosting their immune system with echinacea or using chamomile to calm nerves, herbs work with your dog's body to promote healing from within.

As you move forward with this guide, remember that natural remedies are about more than just treating ailments—they're about fostering a holistic, balanced approach to your dog's overall well-being. The information you'll find here is designed to give you the confidence to integrate herbal remedies into your dog's life in harmony with their unique needs. Whether you're just starting out or have already dabbled in natural care, this book will serve as a comprehensive resource, guiding you toward a healthier, happier life for your beloved pet.

Foundations of Canine Herbalism

CHAPTER 1

"Herbs have been used for centuries to treat animals, including dogs, and they remain a safe and effective option when administered appropriately." — Richard H. Pitcairn

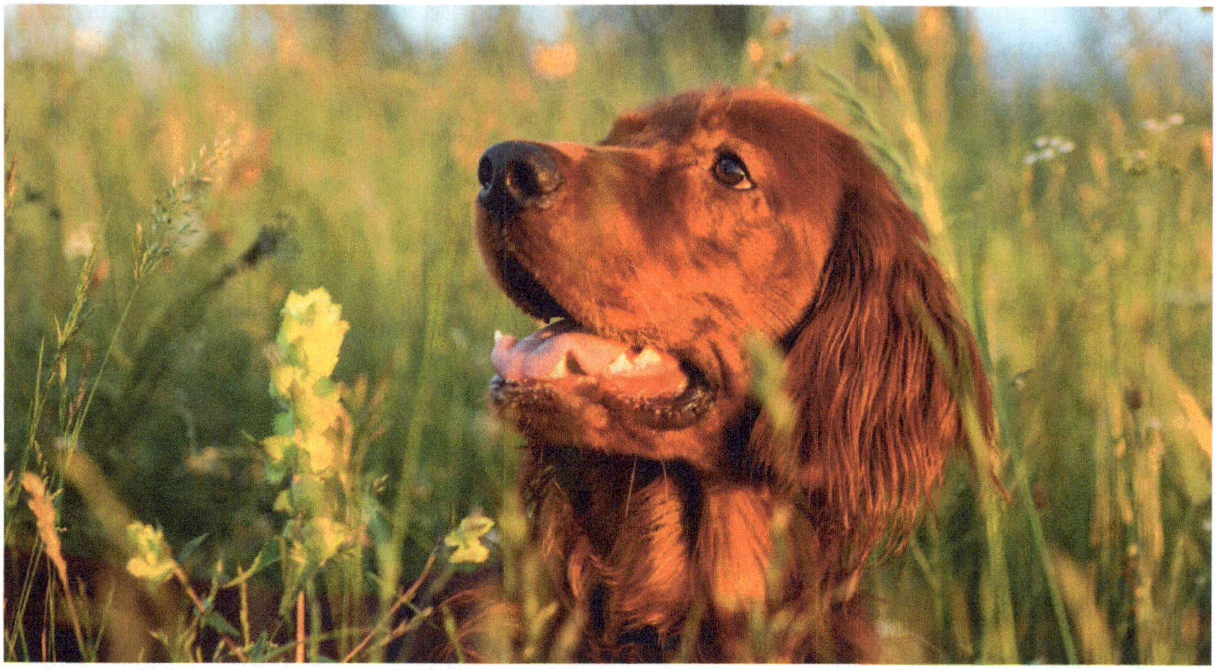

Herbal medicine has been used for centuries, but did you know it's just as effective for dogs as it is for humans? Herbs work with your dog's body, supporting natural healing processes without the harsh side effects often seen in pharmaceuticals. Unlike synthetic drugs that target symptoms, herbs help restore balance in a more holistic way.

In this chapter, you'll learn the basics of herbalism for dogs—how herbs interact with their bodies and why it's important to approach them as medicines, not just supplements. We'll also cover how to use herbs safely, including dosing tips and what to watch out for in terms of side effects. Most importantly, you'll see why it's crucial to collaborate with your veterinarian when exploring herbal remedies for your dog's health. By the end, you'll have the knowledge to begin safely incorporating herbs into your dog's wellness routine.

THE BASICS OF HERBAL MEDICINE

Herbal medicine has been used for over 5,000 years, with around 80% of the global population still relying on plant-based remedies for primary healthcare. Herbalism is more than just a natural alternative; it taps into nature's pharmacy, using the healing power of plants to promote balance and wellness. For dogs, herbs offer a safe and effective way to support health, from boosting the immune system to reducing inflammation and fostering long-term healing and vitality.

What is Herbalism?

Herbalism is the practice of using plants and plant extracts to promote health, prevent disease, and treat various ailments. This ancient form of medicine has been utilized by cultures around the world for thousands of years. In the context of canine health, herbalism involves selecting specific herbs that have been shown to support a dog's body in healing and maintaining balance.

When you think of herbal medicine, you might picture a shelf lined with bottles of dried herbs, tinctures, and capsules. Each of these products represents a piece of nature's pharmacy, offering a range of benefits from calming anxiety to boosting immune function. But herbalism is more than just taking herbs in a pill form. It's about understanding the synergy between plants and the body, recognizing that herbs work holistically—supporting the body's natural processes rather than simply masking symptoms.

How Herbs Work in the Body

Herbs interact with the body in unique and complex ways. Unlike synthetic drugs, which often target a specific symptom or disease process, herbs tend to work more broadly, supporting multiple systems in the body simultaneously. For example, an herb like echinacea not only boosts the immune system but also has anti-inflammatory and antiviral properties, making it a versatile remedy for various conditions.

When it comes to your dog's health, herbs can play a significant role in maintaining balance. They can help support the immune system, improve digestion, reduce inflammation, and even promote mental well-being. The active compounds in herbs, such as alkaloids, flavonoids, and essential oils, interact with the body's cells and tissues, encouraging natural healing processes. For instance, turmeric, a common herb used in both human and canine herbalism, contains curcumin—a compound known for its powerful anti-inflammatory and antioxidant properties. When administered correctly, turmeric can help reduce joint pain in dogs with arthritis and protect their cells from oxidative stress.

It's important to understand that herbs are not a quick fix. They work gradually, allowing the body to heal and strengthen over time. This makes them ideal for chronic conditions or for maintaining long-term health. However, because herbs are potent, they must be used with care, especially when it comes to determining the appropriate dosage and monitoring for any adverse effects.

The Difference Between Medicinal Herbs and Supplements

You might be wondering how herbs differ from the supplements you see at pet stores or online. While both herbs and supplements can be beneficial, there are key differences between the two. Supplements are typically isolated nutrients, such as vitamins or minerals, that are added to a dog's diet to fill nutritional gaps. For example, a supplement might contain a concentrated dose of omega-3 fatty acids to support your dog's skin and coat health.

Herbs, on the other hand, are whole plants or plant parts (like leaves, roots, or flowers) that contain a wide range of active compounds. These compounds work together to produce a therapeutic effect, often addressing multiple aspects of health simultaneously. For instance, milk thistle is an herb commonly used in canine herbalism to support liver function. It contains silymarin, a compound that helps protect liver cells from damage, promotes regeneration, and has antioxidant properties.

Unlike supplements, which often focus on providing a specific nutrient, herbs work more holistically. They don't just supply a single nutrient but rather offer a complex array of compounds that can influence various body systems. This holistic approach can be particularly beneficial in addressing chronic conditions where multiple factors are at play.

SAFETY CONSIDERATIONS

As powerful as herbs can be, it's crucial to approach canine herbalism with caution. Not all herbs are safe for dogs, and even safe herbs must be used correctly to avoid potential side effects. In this section, we'll explore the key safety considerations to keep in mind when using herbal medicine for your dog.

Herbs Safe for Dogs and Toxic Herbs to Avoid

One of the most important aspects of canine herbalism is knowing which herbs are safe and which should be avoided. While many herbs that are beneficial for humans are also safe for dogs, some can be toxic and even deadly to our furry friends.

Safe herbs for dogs include chamomile, known for its calming effects and ability to soothe digestive upset; ginger, which can help with nausea and improve digestion; and calendula, which has anti-inflammatory properties and promotes wound healing. These herbs are generally well-tolerated by dogs and can be used in various forms, such as teas, tinctures, or topical applications.

However, certain herbs should never be given to dogs. For example, garlic, though beneficial for humans, can be toxic to dogs in large quantities, leading to gastrointestinal upset and damage to red blood cells. Similarly, herbs like pennyroyal and wormwood are highly toxic and should be avoided entirely, as they contain compounds that can cause severe harm, including liver damage, seizures, or even death.

To ensure the safety of the herbs you use, always thoroughly research their effects and consult with a veterinarian experienced in herbal medicine. This will help you avoid toxic options and use herbs effectively for your dog's specific needs.

Understanding Dosage and Administration

Determining the correct dosage of an herb for your dog is essential for both safety and efficacy. Unlike pharmaceutical drugs, which often have standardized dosages, herbal medicine requires a more individualized approach. Factors such as your dog's size, age, and overall health must be considered when determining the appropriate dose.

In general, the dosage of an herb is often calculated based on your dog's weight. A common method is to start with a low dose and gradually increase it, monitoring your dog for any adverse reactions. For example, if you're using a tincture of echinacea to support your dog's immune system, you might start with a small dose, such as 0.1 milliliters per pound of body weight, administered once or twice a day.

It's also important to consider the form of the herb you're using. Herbs can be administe-red in various forms, including dried powders, tinctures, teas, or capsules. Each form has its own considerations when it comes to dosage. For instance, tinctures are more con-centrated than teas, so a smaller dose is typically required.

Proper administration is equally important. Some herbs can be mixed into your dog's food, while others may need to be given separately. If your dog is resistant to taking herbs, you may need to get creative with administration, such as hiding the herb in a treat or using a syringe to administer a liquid tincture.

Recognizing Side Effects and When to Seek Veterinary Care

While herbs are generally safe when used correctly, they can cause side effects, particularly if given in too high a dose or for an extended period. Common side effects may include gastrointestinal upset, such as vomiting or diarrhea, especially if your dog is sensitive to the herb or if the dosage is too high.

It's crucial to monitor your dog closely when introducing a new herb into their routine. If you notice any signs of discomfort, such as excessive drooling, lethargy, or changes in appetite, it's essential to stop the herb and consult with your veterinarian. In some cases, side effects may be mild and resolve on their own once the herb is discontinued. However, more severe reactions, such as difficulty breathing, swelling, or seizures, require immediate veterinary attention.

Before adding any herbal remedies to your dog's diet or care routine, it's essential to consult with a veterinarian, preferably one with holistic training or expertise in herbal medicine, as not all vets are familiar with herbal interactions and dosing. Every dog is different, and what benefits one may not be appropriate for another. Your veterinarian can guide you on the safest and most effective approach for your dog's individual health needs. Additionally, be mindful of potential interactions between herbs and other medications your dog may be taking. For example, if your dog is on a blood-thinning medication, herbs like ginkgo biloba or garlic could increase the risk of bleeding. Always inform your veterinarian about any herbs you're using or planning to use so they can help you avoid potential interactions and ensure the safety of your dog's treatment plan.

WORKING WITH YOUR VETERINARIAN

One of the most important aspects of using herbal medicine for your dog is working closely with your veterinarian. While herbs can be a powerful tool for promoting health and healing, they should be used as part of a comprehensive approach to your dog's care, not as a replacement for conventional veterinary treatment.

Integrating Herbal Medicine with Conventional Veterinary Treatments

Herbal medicine can complement conventional veterinary treatments, offering additional support and enhancing the overall effectiveness of your dog's care. For example, if your dog is undergoing treatment for a chronic condition like arthritis, herbs such as turmeric or boswellia can be used alongside prescribed medications to reduce inflammation and pain, potentially allowing for lower doses of pharmaceuticals and reducing the risk of side effects.

When integrating herbal medicine with conventional treatments, communication with your veterinarian is key. Share your interest in using herbs with your vet and work together to develop a treatment plan that incorporates both herbal and conventional therapies. Your vet can help you determine which herbs are appropriate for your dog's condition, how to dose them safely, and how to monitor your dog for any potential interactions or side effects.

It's also important to have realistic expectations about what herbal medicine can achieve. While herbs can provide significant benefits, they are not a cure-all and may not be sufficient on their own for treating serious conditions. In many cases, herbs are most effective when used as part of a broader treatment plan that includes dietary changes, lifestyle modifications, and conventional medical care.

Communicating with Holistic Vets

If you're interested in exploring herbal medicine more deeply, you may want to seek out a holistic veterinarian who specializes in integrative medicine. Holistic vets are trained in both conventional veterinary medicine and alternative therapies, including herbal medicine, acupuncture, and nutrition.

Working with a holistic vet can provide you with a more comprehensive approach to your dog's care, combining the best of both worlds. A holistic vet can help you identify the underlying causes of your dog's health issues and develop a personalized treatment plan that includes herbal remedies, dietary recommendations, and other natural therapies.

When communicating with a holistic vet, be sure to discuss your goals and concerns openly. Whether you're looking to manage a chronic condition, support your dog's overall wellness, or explore alternatives to conventional medications, a holistic vet can guide you in choosing the right herbs and treatments for your dog's unique needs.

THE BOTTOM LINE

In this chapter, you've learned the basics of herbal medicine for dogs. We explored how herbs can work with your dog's body to promote healing and balance, not just as supplements but as powerful natural remedies. You now understand that herbalism offers a different approach from pharmaceutical drugs, focusing on supporting the body's own healing processes.

We also talked about the importance of safety when using herbs. You've seen why proper dosing, administration, and monitoring for side effects are critical. Plus, working closely with your veterinarian ensures your dog gets the best care, especially when combining herbs with other treatments.

In the next chapter, we'll dive into some specific herbs that are safe and effective for dogs. You'll discover how these herbs can target different health issues, from digestive support to calming anxiety. By the end, you'll be ready to choose the right herbs for your dog's unique needs. Let's keep exploring!

Essential Herbs for Dogs

CHAPTER 2

"Integrating herbs into your dog's diet can help address a variety of health issues and support their body's natural ability to heal." – Mary L. Wulff

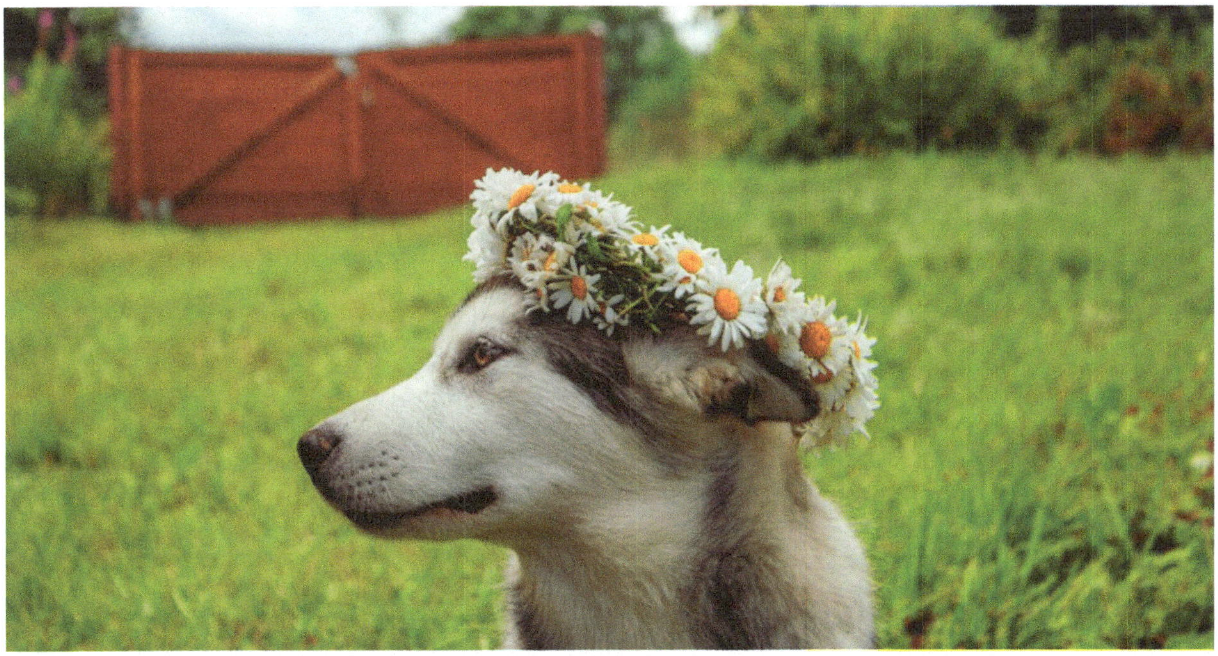

Did you know that some of the most common plants in your garden could be natural remedies for your dog's health? Imagine being able to soothe your dog's upset stomach with chamomile or boost their immune system with echinacea. You'd have a first-aid kit right in your backyard.

In this chapter, you'll learn how to identify herbs that are not only safe but beneficial for dogs. We'll cover how these herbs work, their health benefits, and the right doses for your furry friend. You'll also get a guide on how to grow your own medicinal herb garden so you always have fresh remedies on hand. Finally, we'll dive into detailed profiles of the top 20 healing herbs, explaining exactly how to use each one.

By the end of this chapter, you'll know which herbs can improve your dog's well-being and how to integrate them into their routine.

INTRODUCTION TO CANINE-FRIENDLY HERBS

When it comes to the health and well-being of your dog, you want to ensure that you're doing everything possible to give them a happy, healthy life. You carefully select their food, provide them with exercise, and ensure they get regular vet check-ups. But have you ever considered the potential of incorporating herbs into their routine? Herbs, when used correctly, can be a powerful addition to your dog's health regimen, providing natural support for various conditions and boosting their overall well-being.

What Makes an Herb Beneficial for Dogs?

Not all herbs are created equal, especially when it comes to our furry companions. While some herbs offer tremendous health benefits, others can be harmful or even toxic to dogs. So, what exactly makes an herb beneficial for dogs?

Safety First: Understanding Toxicity and Dosage

The first criterion for determining whether an herb is beneficial for dogs is its safety. Some herbs, such as garlic and onions, are well-known for their toxicity in dogs. Others, like chamomile and ginger, are widely recognized for their safety and effectiveness when used correctly. Understanding the dosage is crucial, as even safe herbs can cause adverse effects if given in excessive amounts. Always start with small doses and consult with your veterinarian, especially if your dog is pregnant, nursing, or on medication.

The Herb's Action: How It Helps

The effectiveness of an herb largely depends on its active constituents and how these components interact with your dog's body. For example, anti-inflammatory herbs like turmeric contain compounds that reduce inflammation and alleviate pain, making them beneficial for dogs with arthritis or other inflammatory conditions. Herbs like milk thistle are known for their detoxifying properties, helping to protect and heal the liver. The action of the herb must align with the specific health needs of your dog to be truly beneficial.

Supporting Overall Health: Adaptogens and Beyond

Some herbs are particularly valuable because they act as adaptogens—substances that help the body resist stressors of all kinds, whether physical, chemical, or biological. Herbs like ashwagandha and Rhodiola fall into this category, helping to improve your dog's resilience to stress and supporting overall well-being. Other herbs can support your dog's immune system, digestion, and even emotional health, making them versatile tools in your natural health toolkit.

Herb Classification by Action

Imagine having a natural remedy for nearly every issue your dog faces—whether it's anxiety, joint pain, or digestive troubles. Herbs, classified by their actions, can help you target these concerns effectively. In this section, you'll learn about different types of herbs and how they work, making it easier to support your dog's health. Whether your dog needs help managing stress, boosting immunity, or easing digestion, these herbs offer powerful, natural solutions.

Adaptogens

Adaptogens are herbs that help the body adapt to stress and restore balance. These herbs are particularly useful for dogs that experience anxiety, nervousness, or physical stress due to illness or aging.

- **Ashwagandha (Withania somnifera):** Known for its calming and strengthening properties, ashwagandha can help manage stress and improve overall vitality in dogs.
- **Rhodiola (Rhodiola rosea):** This herb helps to enhance physical endurance and reduce fatigue, making it ideal for active dogs or those recovering from illness.

Anti-Inflammatories

Anti-inflammatory herbs are crucial for managing conditions like arthritis, allergies, and skin irritations in dogs. These herbs can reduce inflammation and pain, improving your dog's comfort and mobility.

- **Turmeric (Curcuma longa):** A powerful anti-inflammatory, turmeric contains curcumin, which reduces joint pain and inflammation in dogs with arthritis.

- **Ginger (Zingiber officinale):** Ginger not only soothes the digestive system but also has anti-inflammatory properties, making it useful for dogs with arthritis or other inflammatory conditions.

Immune Boosters

Herbs that support the immune system are essential for maintaining your dog's health, particularly during times of stress or illness.

- **Echinacea (Echinacea purpurea):** This herb is well-known for boosting the immune system and can be used to help prevent or treat infections.
- **Astragalus (Astragalus membranaceus):** Astragalus supports immune function and is particularly beneficial for dogs prone to colds or other infections.

Digestive Aids

For dogs with digestive issues, certain herbs can be incredibly helpful in soothing the stomach, improving digestion, and reducing nausea.

- **Chamomile (Matricaria chamomilla):** Chamomile is gentle on the stomach and can help alleviate nausea, gas, and other digestive issues.
- **Peppermint (Mentha piperita):** This herb helps with digestion by reducing gas and easing stomach cramps.

Calming and Relaxing

Herbs that promote relaxation can be particularly helpful for dogs that suffer from anxiety, fear, or hyperactivity.

- **Valerian (Valeriana officinalis):** Valerian is a natural sedative and can be used to calm anxious or hyperactive dogs.
- **Lavender (Lavandula angustifolia):** Known for its soothing aroma, lavender can help reduce stress and anxiety in dogs.

Now that you've explored how herbs are classified by their actions, you're equipped with the knowledge to choose the right ones for your dog's unique needs. Whether it's calming an anxious pup or reducing inflammation, you can now confidently turn to nature's remedies to support your dog's health and well-being.

GROWING YOUR OWN MEDICINAL HERB GARDEN

There's something truly rewarding about growing your own herbs, especially when you know they'll contribute to your dog's health. Cultivating a medicinal herb garden allows you to have fresh, organic herbs at your fingertips, ensuring that your dog gets the best quality possible.

Best Practices for Cultivating Herbs at Home

Whether you have a large garden or just a small windowsill, growing herbs at home is accessible to everyone. Here are some best practices to ensure a thriving herb garden:

Choosing the Right Location

Herbs generally thrive in well-drained soil and require plenty of sunlight—at least 6-8 hours per day. If you're growing herbs indoors, place them near a south-facing window where they can soak up the sun. If outdoor space is available, choose a spot that is sheltered from strong winds but still receives ample light.

Soil Preparation and Planting

Herbs prefer a slightly alkaline to neutral soil pH (6.0-7.5). Before planting, enrich the soil with organic compost to provide essential nutrients. For those planting in containers, use a high-quality potting mix that drains well. Space the herbs according to their needs, as overcrowding can lead to poor growth and disease.

Watering and Care

Most herbs prefer to dry out slightly between waterings, so avoid overwatering, which can lead to root rot. Water the plants early in the day, giving them time to dry before nightfall. Regularly prune the herbs to encourage bushier growth and prevent them from flowering too early, which can reduce their potency.

Harvesting, Drying, and Storing Herbs for Canine Use

Knowing when and how to harvest your herbs is key to ensuring they retain their medicinal properties. Here's how to do it right:

Harvesting

The best time to harvest herbs is in the morning after the dew has dried but before the sun gets too hot. This is when the essential oils are most concentrated in the leaves. Use sharp scissors or pruning shears to cut the herbs, leaving at least a third of the plant intact to encourage regrowth.

Drying

To dry herbs, tie them in small bundles and hang them upside down in a warm, well-ventilated area out of direct sunlight. Alternatively, you can spread them out on a drying rack or use a dehydrator set to a low temperature. The herbs are ready when they crumble easily between your fingers.

Storing

Once dried, store herbs in airtight containers away from light and moisture to preserve their potency. Glass jars with tight-fitting lids are ideal. Label each jar with the name of the herb and the date it was harvested. Properly stored herbs can retain their potency for up to a year.

TOP 20 HEALING HERBS FOR DOGS

Now that you have a good understanding of how to identify beneficial herbs and grow them at home let's delve into the profiles of the top 20 healing herbs for dogs. Each profile includes the herb's scientific name, properties, health benefits, dosage recommendations, and practical applications. This information will help you confidently incorporate these herbs into your dog's routine.

Turmeric (Curcuma longa)

Properties: Anti-inflammatory, antioxidant, anti-cancer.

Health Benefits: Turmeric is renowned for its anti-inflammatory properties, making it highly effective for dogs with arthritis or joint pain. It also has antioxidant properties that help neutralize harmful free radicals in the body, potentially reducing the risk of cancer.

Dosage: Start with 1/8 to 1/4 teaspoon per 10 pounds of body weight, mixed with food. Gradually increase the dosage based on your dog's response.

Applications: Turmeric can be mixed into your dog's food or made into a paste with coconut oil to increase its absorption.

Precaution: Before introducing any herbal remedies to your dog's diet or care routine, always consult with a veterinarian. Each dog is unique, and what works for one may not be suitable for another. Your veterinarian can help determine the best approach for your dog's specific health needs and conditions.

Chamomile (Matricaria chamomilla)

Properties: Anti-inflammatory, calming, digestive aid.

Health Benefits: Chamomile is a gentle herb that soothes the stomach, relieves anxiety and reduces inflammation. It's particularly useful for dogs with digestive issues or those who are anxious or hyperactive.

Dosage: Offer chamomile as a tea or tincture. For tea, steep 1 teaspoon of dried flowers in a cup of hot water, let it cool and give 1-2 teaspoons to small dogs or 1-2 tablespoons to larger dogs.

Applications: Chamomile tea can be added to your dog's water or food. It can also be applied topically to soothe skin irritations.

Precaution: Before introducing any herbal remedies to your dog's diet or care routine, always consult with a veterinarian. Each dog is unique, and what works for one may not be suitable for another. Your veterinarian can help determine the best approach for your dog's specific health needs and conditions.

Milk Thistle (Silybum marianum)

Properties: Liver detoxifier, antioxidant.

Health Benefits: Milk thistle is the go-to herb for supporting liver health in dogs. It helps detoxify the liver, making it beneficial for dogs exposed to toxins or those on long-term medications.

Dosage: Use milk thistle extract or powder, giving 1/4 teaspoon per 20 pounds of body weight daily.

Applications: Mix milk thistle powder into your dog's food, or use a tincture that can be added to water or food.

Precaution: Before introducing any herbal remedies to your dog's diet or care routine, always consult with a veterinarian. Each dog is unique, and what works for one may not be suitable for another. Your veterinarian can help determine the best approach for your dog's specific health needs and conditions.

Ginger (Zingiber officinale)

Properties: Anti-inflammatory, digestive aid, anti-nausea.

Health Benefits: Ginger is excellent for soothing the digestive system, reducing nausea, and alleviating inflammation. It's particularly helpful for dogs with arthritis or those prone to motion sickness.

Dosage: Give 1/4 teaspoon per 10 pounds of body weight, mixed with food. For nausea, you can also offer ginger tea in small amounts.

Applications: Ginger can be added to food or made into tea. It can also be used in homemade dog treats.

Precaution: Before introducing any herbal remedies to your dog's diet or care routine, always consult with a veterinarian. Each dog is unique, and what works for one may not be suitable for another. Your veterinarian can help determine the best approach for your dog's specific health needs and conditions.

Echinacea (Echinacea purpurea)

Properties: Immune booster, anti-inflammatory, antimicrobial

Health Benefits: Echinacea is known for its immune-boosting properties, helping to ward off infections and reduce inflammation. It's especially useful during cold and flu season or when your dog is under stress.

Dosage: Use Echinacea tincture, giving 0.5 ml per 20 pounds of body weight up to twice daily.

Applications: Add Echinacea tincture to your dog's water or food. It can also be used topically to treat minor wounds or skin infections.

Precaution: Before introducing any herbal remedies to your dog's diet or care routine, always consult with a veterinarian. Each dog is unique, and what works for one may not be suitable for another. Your veterinarian can help determine the best approach for your dog's specific health needs and conditions.

Lavender (Lavandula angustifolia)

Properties: Calming, antimicrobial, anti-inflammatory.

Health Benefits: Lavender is a versatile herb that calms anxiety, aids sleep and soothes skin irritations. It's also antimicrobial, making it useful for treating minor wounds or infections.

Dosage: Use lavender essential oil diluted in a carrier oil for topical use, or offer lavender tea (1 teaspoon of dried flowers per cup of water) in small amounts.

Applications: Apply diluted lavender oil to your dog's bedding to help them relax. Lavender tea can be added to water or food.

Precaution: Before introducing any herbal remedies to your dog's diet or care routine, always consult with a veterinarian. Each dog is unique, and what works for one may not be suitable for another. Your veterinarian can help determine the best approach for your dog's specific health needs and conditions.

Peppermint (Mentha piperita)

Properties: Digestive aid, anti-nausea, cooling.

Health Benefits: Peppermint soothes the stomach, reduces nausea, and can be used to cool your dog down on hot days. It's particularly useful for dogs with digestive issues or those that suffer from heat stress.

Dosage: Offer peppermint tea or tincture in small amounts—1/2 teaspoon of tea for small dogs and 1 tablespoon for larger dogs.

Applications: Peppermint tea can be added to your dog's water or food. A few drops of peppermint oil diluted in water can be used as a cooling spray.

Precaution: Before introducing any herbal remedies to your dog's diet or care routine, always consult with a veterinarian. Each dog is unique, and what works for one may not be suitable for another. Your veterinarian can help determine the best approach for your dog's specific health needs and conditions.

Valerian (Valeriana officinalis)

Properties: Sedative, calming.

Health Benefits: Valerian is a natural sedative that helps reduce anxiety and promote sleep. It's particularly useful for dogs that are hyperactive or anxious during storms or fireworks.

Dosage: Use valerian tincture, giving 0.5 ml per 20 pounds of body weight, up to twice daily.

Applications: Add valerian tincture to your dog's water or food, or offer valerian tea (1 teaspoon of dried root per cup of water) in small amounts.

Precaution: Before introducing any herbal remedies to your dog's diet or care routine, always consult with a veterinarian. Each dog is unique, and what works for one may not be suitable for another. Your veterinarian can help determine the best approach for your dog's specific health needs and conditions.

Calendula (Calendula officinalis)

Properties: Antimicrobial, anti-inflammatory, wound healer.

Health Benefits: Calendula is known for its wound-healing properties, making it ideal for treating cuts, scrapes, and other minor injuries. It also has anti-inflammatory and antimicrobial properties.

Dosage: Use calendula tincture or tea for topical application.

Applications: Apply calendula tea or diluted tincture to wounds or skin irritations. Calendula can also be used in homemade salves.

Precaution: Before introducing any herbal remedies to your dog's diet or care routine, always consult with a veterinarian. Each dog is unique, and what works for one may not be suitable for another. Your veterinarian can help determine the best approach for your dog's specific health needs and conditions.

Dandelion (Taraxacum officinale)

Properties: Diuretic, liver detoxifier, digestive aid.

Health Benefits: Dandelion is a gentle diuretic that supports liver health and aids digestion. It's particularly beneficial for dogs with liver issues or those that need gentle detoxification.

Dosage: Give 1/2 teaspoon of dried dandelion root or leaves per 20 pounds of body weight, mixed with food.

Applications: Add dandelion to your dog's food or make tea for a gentle detox.

Precaution: Before introducing any herbal remedies to your dog's diet or care routine, always consult with a veterinarian. Each dog is unique, and what works for one may not be suitable for another. Your veterinarian can help determine the best approach for your dog's specific health needs and conditions.

Marshmallow Root (Althaea officinalis)

Properties: Anti-inflammatory, digestive aid, wound healer.

Health Benefits: Marshmallow root soothes the digestive tract and reduces inflammation, making it useful for dogs with gastrointestinal issues. It also promotes wound healing.

Dosage: Offer marshmallow root tea (1 teaspoon per cup of water) in small amounts, or mix the dried root into food.

Applications: Use marshmallow root tea to soothe an irritated digestive tract or apply it topically to wounds.

Precaution: Before introducing any herbal remedies to your dog's diet or care routine, always consult with a veterinarian. Each dog is unique, and what works for one may not be suitable for another. Your veterinarian can help determine the best approach for your dog's specific health needs and conditions.

Rosemary (Rosmarinus officinalis)

Properties: Antioxidant, antimicrobial, memory booster.

Health Benefits: Rosemary is rich in antioxidants and has antimicrobial properties, making it beneficial for overall health. It's also believed to boost memory and cognitive function in aging dogs.

Dosage: Add a pinch of dried rosemary to your dog's food, or use rosemary essential oil (diluted) for topical application.

Applications: Rosemary can be added to food as a seasoning or used in homemade dog treats. Diluted rosemary oil can be applied to the coat for its antimicrobial benefits.

Precaution: Before introducing any herbal remedies to your dog's diet or care routine, always consult with a veterinarian. Each dog is unique, and what works for one may not be suitable for another. Your veterinarian can help determine the best approach for your dog's specific health needs and conditions.

Thyme (Thymus vulgaris)

Properties: Antimicrobial, antioxidant, digestive aid.

Health Benefits: Thyme is a powerful antimicrobial herb that also supports digestion and boosts the immune system. It's particularly useful for dogs with respiratory issues or those prone to infections.

Dosage: Add a pinch of dried thyme to your dog's food, or offer thyme tea in small amounts.

Applications: Thyme can be used in food, made into tea, or applied topically (diluted) to treat minor infections.

Precaution: Before introducing any herbal remedies to your dog's diet or care routine, always consult with a veterinarian. Each dog is unique, and what works for one may not be suitable for another. Your veterinarian can help determine the best approach for your dog's specific health needs and conditions.

Parsley (Petroselinum crispum)

Properties: Digestive aid, diuretic, breath freshener.

Health Benefits: Parsley supports digestion, acts as a diuretic, and can help freshen your dog's breath. It's a great herb to add to your dog's diet for overall health support.

Dosage: Add 1/4 teaspoon of chopped fresh parsley per 10 pounds of body weight to food.

Applications: Parsley can be chopped and added to your dog's food or used as a breath freshener by offering small amounts directly.

Precaution: Before introducing any herbal remedies to your dog's diet or care routine, always consult with a veterinarian. Each dog is unique, and what works for one may not be suitable for another. Your veterinarian can help determine the best approach for your dog's specific health needs and conditions.

Oregano (Origanum vulgare)

Properties: Antimicrobial, antioxidant, anti-inflammatory.

Health Benefits: Oregano is a potent antimicrobial herb that also has anti-inflammatory and antioxidant properties. It's useful for treating infections and boosting overall health.

Dosage: Add a small pinch of dried oregano to your dog's food, or use oregano oil (diluted) for topical application.

Applications: Oregano can be added to food, used in homemade dog treats, or applied topically (diluted) to treat infections.

Precaution: Before introducing any herbal remedies to your dog's diet or care routine, always consult with a veterinarian. Each dog is unique, and what works for one may not be suitable for another. Your veterinarian can help determine the best approach for your dog's specific health needs and conditions.

Licorice Root (Glycyrrhiza glabra)

Properties: Anti-inflammatory, immune booster, digestive aid.

Health Benefits: Licorice root is a powerful anti-inflammatory that also supports the immune system and aids digestion. It's particularly useful for dogs with allergies or autoimmune conditions.

Dosage: Use licorice root powder, giving 1/4 teaspoon per 10 pounds of body weight, mixed with food.

Applications: Licorice root can be added to food, made into tea, or used in homemade dog treats.

Precaution: Before introducing any herbal remedies to your dog's diet or care routine, always consult with a veterinarian. Each dog is unique, and what works for one may not be suitable for another. Your veterinarian can help determine the best approach for your dog's specific health needs and conditions.

Basil (Ocimum basilicum)

Properties: Antioxidant, anti-inflammatory, antimicrobial.

Health Benefits: Basil is a versatile herb that offers antioxidant, anti-inflammatory, and antimicrobial benefits. It's particularly useful for boosting overall health and treating minor infections.

Dosage: Add a small pinch of fresh or dried basil to your dog's food.

Applications: Basil can be added to food, used in homemade dog treats, or made into tea.

Precaution: Before introducing any herbal remedies to your dog's diet or care routine, always consult with a veterinarian. Each dog is unique, and what works for one may not be suitable for another. Your veterinarian can help determine the best approach for your dog's specific health needs and conditions.

Sage (Salvia officinalis)

Properties: Antimicrobial, antioxidant, anti-inflammatory.

Health Benefits: Sage is known for its antimicrobial and antioxidant properties, making it useful for treating infections and supporting overall health. It's also believed to improve cognitive function in aging dogs.

Dosage: Add a small pinch of dried sage to your dog's food, or offer sage tea in small amounts.

Applications: Sage can be added to food, used in homemade dog treats, or applied topically (diluted) to treat infections.

Precaution: Before introducing any herbal remedies to your dog's diet or care routine, always consult with a veterinarian. Each dog is unique, and what works for one may not be suitable for another. Your veterinarian can help determine the best approach for your dog's specific health needs and conditions.

Catnip (Nepeta cataria)

Properties: Calming, digestive aid, antimicrobial.

Health Benefits: While best known for its effects on cats, catnip can also benefit dogs by calming anxiety, soothing the stomach, and providing antimicrobial support.

Dosage: Offer catnip tea or tincture in small amounts or mix dried catnip into food.

Applications: Catnip can be used as a calming agent, digestive aid, or antimicrobial treatment.

Precaution: Before introducing any herbal remedies to your dog's diet or care routine, always consult with a veterinarian. Each dog is unique, and what works for one may not be suitable for another. Your veterinarian can help determine the best approach for your dog's specific health needs and conditions.

Nettle (Urtica dioica)

Properties: Anti-inflammatory, immune booster, diuretic.

Health Benefits: Nettle is a nutrient-rich herb that reduces inflammation, supports the immune system, and acts as a natural diuretic. It's particularly useful for dogs with allergies or inflammatory conditions.

Dosage: Add 1/4 teaspoon of dried nettle per 10 pounds of body weight to food.

Applications: Nettle can be added to food, made into tea, or used in homemade dog treats.

Precaution: Before introducing any herbal remedies to your dog's diet or care routine, always consult with a veterinarian. Each dog is unique, and what works for one may not be suitable for another. Your veterinarian can help determine the best approach for your dog's specific health needs and conditions. Always consult a veterinarian before giving herbal medication to your pets. This is important because individual pets may react differently to herbs, and certain health conditions or medications may interact with herbal treatments. Your veterinarian can provide guidance on safe usage, proper dosages, and potential side effects tailored to your pet's specific needs.

THE BOTTOM LINE

In this chapter, you've learned about the powerful healing herbs that can boost your dog's health. We've explored how to identify which herbs are safe and beneficial, from adaptogens that help with stress to immune boosters that keep your dog strong. You've also discovered the top 20 healing herbs and how each one can make a difference in your dog's well-being. Whether it's treating inflammation or supporting digestion, these herbs offer natural solutions. And for those wanting to grow their own medicinal garden, we covered how to plant, harvest, and store these herbs at home.

Now that you have a solid foundation on essential herbs, it's time to put that knowledge into action. In the next chapter, we'll dive into how to use these remedies in your dog's daily life. You'll find practical tips on incorporating herbal care into meals, grooming, and more. It's all about making these natural treatments a part of your dog's routine. Let's take that next step together!

How to Use Herbal Medicine in Yours's Dog Daily

CHAPTER 3

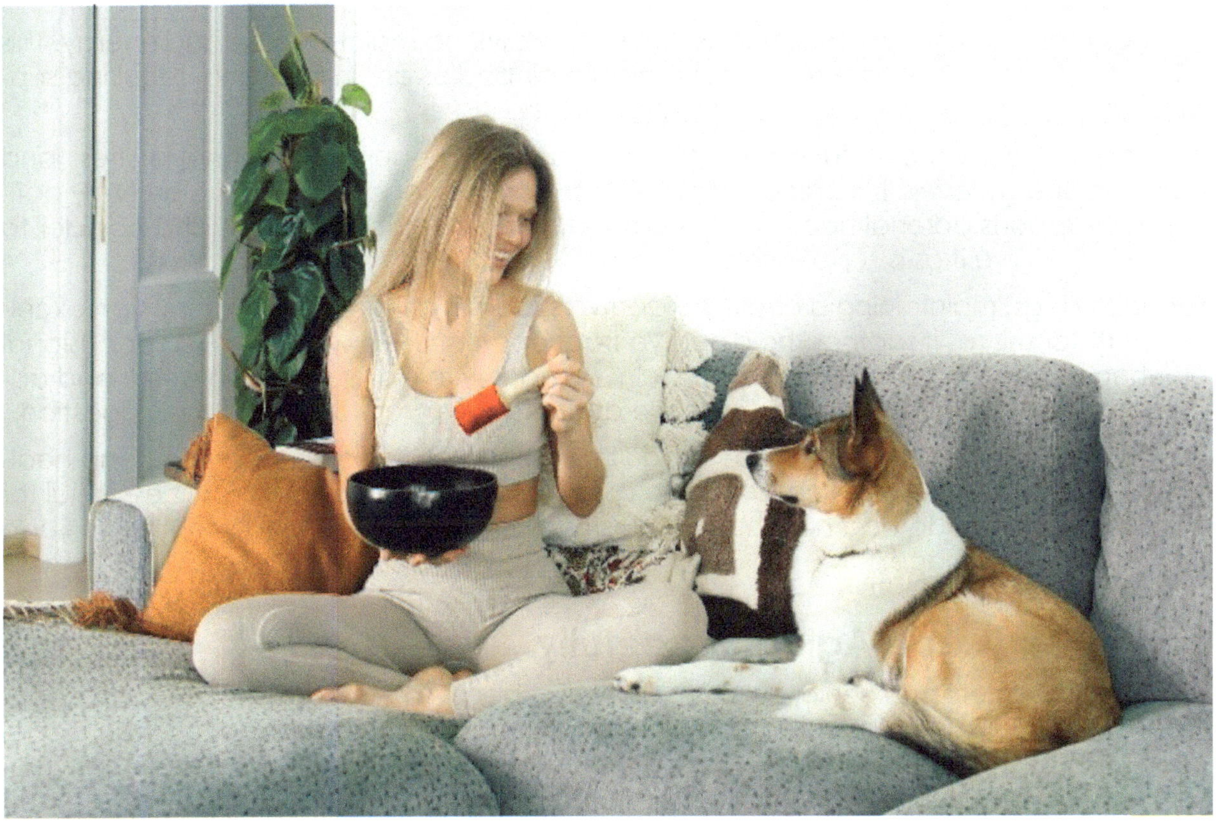

HERBAL SUPPORT FOR LIFE STAGES

Just as the nutritional needs of dogs change as they grow, so do their herbal needs. Understanding how to tailor your dog's herbal regimen to their life stage ensures they receive the best possible care at every phase of life.

Puppies and Growing Dogs

Puppies are bundles of energy, curiosity, and growth. During this critical stage, their bodies are developing rapidly, and their immune systems are still maturing. Herbs can play a vital role in supporting this growth, strengthening their immune system, and ensuring they develop into healthy adults.

Echinacea is an excellent herb for puppies, known for its immune-boosting properties. Introducing echinacea into a puppy's routine can help them ward off common illnesses and infections as they explore their environment. You might mix a small amount of echinacea tincture into their food or water, especially during the cold and flu season.

Licorice root is another beneficial herb for puppies, particularly for its anti-inflammatory properties. It can soothe digestive issues that are common in young dogs, especially as they transition to solid foods. A little licorice root tea added to their diet can make a significant difference in their digestive comfort.

As puppies grow, their joints and bones are under a lot of stress. Alfalfa is rich in minerals like calcium and can support healthy bone development. Adding dried alfalfa to their food can help ensure they're getting the nutrients they need for strong bones and joints.

Adult Dogs and Their Specific Needs

As dogs reach adulthood, their needs shift from growth to maintenance and energy. This is the stage where they are most active, and their bodies are in full swing, requiring support for stamina, muscle health, and overall vitality.

Ashwagandha is a powerful adaptogen that can help adult dogs manage stress and maintain energy levels. It's particularly useful for working dogs or those who are very active, as it supports adrenal health and resilience. You can add ashwagandha powder to their food or give it as a supplement.

For adult dogs, maintaining a healthy digestive system is crucial. Slippery elm is an excellent herb for this, as it soothes the digestive tract and can help with issues like occasional diarrhea or constipation. Mixing slippery elm powder with water to form a paste and adding it to your dog's food can be a gentle and effective way to support their digestion.

Hawthorn is another fantastic herb for adult dogs, particularly for supporting heart health. This herb strengthens the heart muscle and improves circulation, which is essential for active dogs. You can add hawthorn berries or a tincture to your dog's routine to keep their heart in top shape.

Senior Dogs and Aging Gracefully

As your dog enters their senior years, their bodies begin to slow down. Their joints might stiffen, their energy levels decrease, and they become more susceptible to chronic conditions. Herbs can provide gentle support during this time, helping your dog age gracefully and stay comfortable.

Turmeric becomes even more valuable in a senior dog's regimen. Its anti-inflammatory properties can ease joint pain and stiffness, making it a must-have for older dogs prone to arthritis. A daily dose of turmeric mixed with a bit of black pepper and healthy fat, like coconut oil, can provide significant relief.

Ginkgo biloba is another herb that can benefit senior dogs, particularly for cognitive health. As dogs age, they may experience cognitive decline, similar to dementia in humans. Ginkgo biloba improves blood circulation to the brain, supporting mental clarity and reducing the symptoms of cognitive dysfunction. You can give it in tincture form or as a dried herb.

Devil's claw is a potent anti-inflammatory and pain reliever, making it ideal for managing chronic pain in older dogs. It's particularly useful for dogs suffering from arthritis or hip dysplasia. Adding devil's claw to your dog's diet can help them stay active and comfortable in their golden years.

Dandelion root is beneficial for supporting liver and kidney function, which is crucial as dogs age. These organs often require additional support to process toxins effectively. A daily dose of dandelion root tea or powder can help keep these organs functioning optimally.

Always consult your veterinarian before introducing any herbs to your dog's diet, especially if they are on medication or have pre-existing conditions. Herbal remedies can interact with medications or cause side effects if not used properly.

PREPARING HERBAL TEAS, TINCTURES, AND POWDERS

Now that you understand which herbs are beneficial for your dog at different life stages, the next step is learning how to prepare and administer them. The goal is to make these remedies as effective and palatable as possible.

Techniques for Brewing and Mixing Herbs

Herbal teas are one of the easiest ways to administer herbs to your dog. To make a basic herbal tea, you'll need dried herbs and hot water. For instance, to brew a chamomile tea:

Measure the herbs: Use about one teaspoon of dried chamomile for every cup of water.

Boil the water: Bring the water to a rolling boil, then remove it from heat.

Steep the herbs: Pour the hot water over the herbs and let them steep for 5-10 minutes. The longer you steep, the stronger the tea.

Cool and strain: Allow the tea to cool to room temperature, then strain out the herbs.

You can then add this tea to your dog's water bowl or mix it with their food. For dogs who are finicky, consider mixing the tea with a bit of broth to enhance the flavor.

Tinctures are another effective way to administer herbs, especially those that your dog might not enjoy in their food. Tinctures are concentrated herbal extracts made by soaking herbs in alcohol or glycerin. For dogs, glycerin-based tinctures are often preferred as they're alcohol-free and taste sweeter. To make a tincture:

Fill a jar with herbs: Use dried or fresh herbs and pack them into a glass jar.

Add glycerin: Pour vegetable glycerin over the herbs until they're fully submerged.

Seal and shake: Seal the jar and shake it daily, keeping it in a cool, dark place for 4-6 weeks.

Strain and store: After the steeping period, strain the herbs out and store the tincture in a dark glass bottle.

Tinctures are highly concentrated, so you'll only need to give your dog a few drops at a time. Add the drops to their food or water, or administer them directly into their mouth.

How to Administer Herbs to Picky Eaters

Administering herbs to a picky eater can be challenging, but with a few tricks, you can ensure your dog gets the benefits without the struggle. Here are some strategies:

Mix with favorite foods: Combine the herbs with foods your dog loves, such as peanut butter, cheese, or yogurt. The strong flavors of these foods can mask the taste of the herbs.

Create herbal capsules: For dogs who refuse herbs in any form, consider making your own herbal capsules. You can fill empty gelatin capsules with powdered herbs and give them as you would a pill.

Use broth or gravy: Mix herbs with a small amount of broth or gravy to make them more palatable. This works well for teas and powders.

Herbal-infused treats: You can make homemade dog treats infused with herbs. This way, your dog will associate the herbs with a tasty reward.

By being creative and patient, you can find the right method that works for your dog.

Topical Applications: Salves, Oils, and Poultices

Herbal remedies are not limited to teas or tinctures; many herbs are just as effective when used externally. Topical applications such as salves, oils, and poultices offer powerful healing solutions for skin issues, wounds, joint pain, and more. These methods work by delivering the healing properties of herbs directly to the affected area, making them an excellent choice for localized treatment. Here's a closer look at how you can use herbs externally to promote healing and well-being.

Herbal Salves

Salves are thick ointments created by combining infused oils with beeswax. They are highly effective for treating minor cuts, scrapes, burns, dry skin, and even insect bites. Salves create a protective barrier over the skin, allowing the herbs to work their magic while sealing in moisture and keeping contaminants out. To make an herbal salve, follow these steps:

Infuse the Oil: Begin by placing dried herbs of your choice (such as calendula, comfrey, or lavender) in a clean jar and covering them with a carrier oil, such as olive, coconut, or almond oil. Let the mixture infuse for 4-6 weeks in a warm, sunny spot, shaking the jar occasionally to encourage infusion. If you need the salve sooner, you can speed up the process by gently heating the herbs and oil in a double boiler for a few hours.

Strain and Heat: Once the oil is fully infused, strain out the herbs using a cheesecloth or fine mesh strainer. Next, gently heat the infused oil in a pan and add beeswax. Use roughly one ounce of beeswax for every cup of oil. Stir until the beeswax melts completely.

Pour and Cool: Pour the melted mixture into small tins or glass jars and allow it to cool. As the salve cools, it will solidify into a soft, balm-like consistency. Once set, the salve is ready to use. It can be stored in a cool, dark place and will typically last for several months.

Some popular herbs used in salves include calendula, known for its soothing, anti-inflammatory properties, and comfrey, which promotes cell regeneration and is particularly beneficial for healing wounds, sprains, and bruises.

Herbal Oils

Herbal oils are essentially infused oils that have not been thickened with beeswax. These oils are incredibly versatile and can be used for a variety of purposes, including massage, skincare, and treating sore muscles or inflamed joints. They are simple to make and can be applied directly to the skin or incorporated into other products like lotions or shampoos.

For instance, calendula oil is well-known for its ability to soothe irritated skin and reduce inflammation, making it ideal for conditions such as eczema, psoriasis, or diaper rash. Comfrey oil can be massaged into achy joints or bruises to encourage faster healing. Additionally, lavender oil is perfect for relaxation, and massaging it into your temples or neck can help relieve tension headaches.

Poultices

A poultice is a quick and effective way to deliver the healing properties of herbs directly to the skin. Unlike salves or oils, poultices are made from fresh or dried herbs that are crushed or moistened to create a paste. This herbal paste is then applied directly to the skin and covered with a cloth or bandage to keep it in place. Poultices are particularly useful for drawing out toxins, soothing infections, or reducing swelling from bites, stings, and other injuries. For example, Broadleaf plantain, a common "weed" found in many yards, can be used to make a poultice that draws out venom from insect stings or soothes skin irritations. To make a plantain poultice:

- Crush fresh plantain leaves to release their juices.
- Apply the crushed leaves directly to the affected area.
- Cover with a clean cloth or bandage and leave it in place for 15-30 minutes.
- Reapply as needed until the irritation subsides.

Poultices made from herbs like comfrey and ginger can help reduce inflammation and relieve pain in sore muscles or arthritic joints.

Customizing Your Herbal Treatments

When using herbs topically, it's essential to tailor your remedies to your specific needs. Different herbs offer unique benefits, so it's important to choose the right one for your situation. Whether you're dealing with a stubborn skin condition or sore muscles, there is likely an herbal salve, oil, or poultice that can provide relief.

As always, it's a good idea to do a patch test before using any new herbal remedy on a larger area of skin, especially if you have sensitive skin or are prone to allergic reactions. With proper use, these herbal treatments can become powerful tools in your natural healing routine. Also, always consult with a veterinarian before administering any herbal medication to your pets. While these herbs offer potential health benefits, every dog is unique, and some herbs may not be suitable for certain conditions, breeds, or existing medications. A veterinarian can provide personalized guidance and ensure your pet's safety.

THE BOTTOM LINE

In this chapter, you've learned how to make herbal remedies a natural part of your dog's daily routine. By now, you understand that herbs are not just for treating illness—they're a powerful way to maintain your dog's overall health. Whether it's a calming tea for stress or a tincture to boost immunity, herbs can easily fit into your dog's life, no matter their age.

We've also explored how your dog's herbal needs change with each life stage. Puppies need gentle support as they grow, while adult dogs benefit from herbs that promote vitality. For senior dogs, herbs can help with joint support and overall comfort. You're now equipped with simple, daily routines to keep your dog healthy from puppyhood to their golden years.

On the practical side, we covered how to prepare herbal teas, tinctures, and powders. You now have easy instructions to create these remedies at home, plus tips for getting even the pickiest eater to enjoy them.

As you move to the next chapter, we'll dive deeper into specific issues. The next chapter will guide you through treating everyday problems like digestive upset, anxiety, and skin issues. You'll discover which herbs work best for these conditions and how to safely use them. Get ready to tackle the most common health challenges with the knowledge you've gained.

Common Canine Ailments and Herbal Treatments

CHAPTER 4

"Many common canine ailments, including digestive upsets, respiratory conditions, and skin disorders, can benefit from herbal approaches that are tailored to the specific needs of the animal." – Gregory L. Tilford

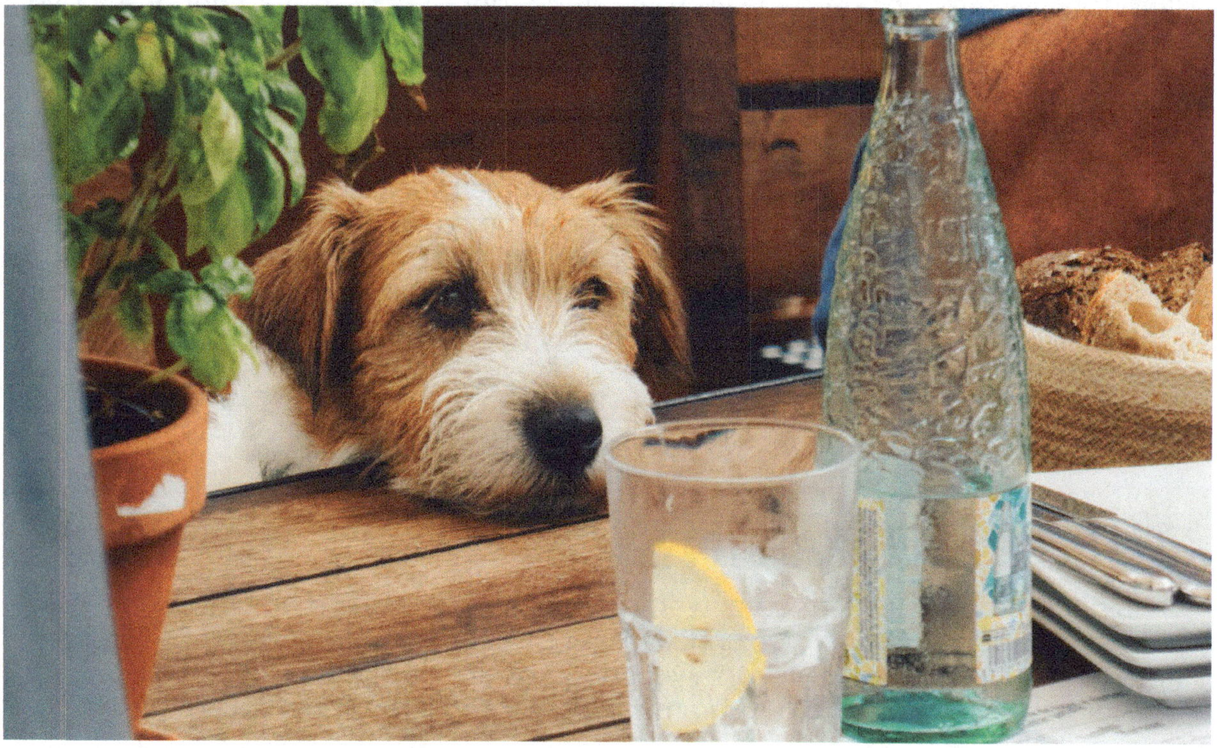

You love your dog, and you'd do anything to ensure they live a healthy, happy life. But sometimes, despite your best efforts, your furry friend might encounter health challenges that leave you feeling worried and uncertain. When those inevitable bumps in the road appear, you want to be prepared with safe, effective, and natural solutions that align with your commitment to holistic care. That's where the power of herbal treatments comes in—a gentle yet powerful way to support your dog's health, addressing common ailments with remedies straight from nature.

In this chapter, you'll discover how to harness the healing power of herbs to tackle a range of health issues that dogs often face. From itchy skin and digestive troubles to anxiety and joint pain, herbal remedies offer a way to treat these problems without relying solely on pharmaceuticals. Not only do these natural treatments often come with fewer side effects, but they also promote overall wellness by supporting your dog's body as a whole. Whether you're dealing with chronic conditions or occasional flare-ups, you're about to learn how to become your dog's best advocate for natural health. Let's dive in.

SKIN AND COAT ISSUES

Your dog's skin and coat are not just a beauty factor—they're vital indicators of overall health. When skin issues arise, such as itching, rashes, or hot spots, it can be distressing for both you and your pet. These problems are often a sign that something deeper is amiss, whether it's an allergy, an imbalance in diet, or a reaction to environmental factors. Fortunately, nature offers a range of herbal remedies that can soothe these symptoms and address the underlying causes.

Herbs for Itching, Rashes, and Allergies

Itching and rashes can drive your dog—and you—crazy. Persistent scratching not only irritates the skin further but can lead to secondary infections. To get to the root of the issue, it's essential to consider what might be triggering the problem, such as fleas, food allergies, or even stress. However, while you're investigating the cause, there are several herbs you can use to provide immediate relief.

Chamomile is one of the most soothing herbs for the skin. Known for its anti-inflammatory and calming properties, chamomile can be used as a topical wash to relieve itching and reduce redness. Simply brew a strong chamomile tea, let it cool, and apply it to the affected areas with a soft cloth. The gentle astringent qualities of chamomile help to dry out rashes while reducing discomfort.

Another powerful herb is calendula. Often referred to as "nature's antiseptic," calendula is excellent for treating skin irritations and infections. It speeds up the healing of cuts, scrapes, and rashes, and it's especially effective when used in an ointment or salve. You can make a simple calendula oil by infusing the dried flowers in olive oil for several weeks, then straining and applying the oil directly to irritated skin. For dogs suffering from allergies, nettles can be a game-changer. Nettles are rich in histamine-lowering compounds, which makes them particularly useful for reducing allergic reactions. When given internally, either as a tincture or mixed into food, nettles can help reduce the overall sensitivity to allergens.

Before introducing any herbal remedies to your dog's diet or care routine, always consult with a veterinarian. Each dog is unique, and what works for one may not be suitable for another. Your veterinarian can help determine the best approach for your dog's specific health needs and conditions.

Remedies for Hot Spots, Eczema, and Dandruff

Hot spots—those red, inflamed areas that seem to appear out of nowhere—are often caused by excessive licking, scratching, or biting. These lesions can escalate quickly, becoming painful and prone to infection. Eczema, which manifests as dry, flaky, or greasy patches, and dandruff, caused by dry skin, are other common skin issues that can make your dog uncomfortable.

One of the best herbal remedies for hot spots is aloe vera. Aloe's cooling gel not only soothes the inflamed area but also acts as a barrier, preventing your dog from further irritating the spot. You can apply pure aloe vera gel directly to the hot spot several times a day to promote healing.

For eczema and dandruff, burdock root is highly effective. Burdock is a blood purifier that helps to eliminate toxins from the body, making it a great herb for skin conditions linked to internal imbalances. You can use burdock root in tincture form or as a tea added to your dog's food to improve skin health from the inside out.

Oatmeal is another wonderful remedy, especially for dry, itchy skin and dandruff. An oatmeal bath can work wonders, providing instant relief from itching and soothing irritated skin. Grind plain, unsweetened oatmeal into a fine powder and add it to a warm bath. Let your dog soak for 10-15 minutes, which will help to moisturize and calm the skin. Before adding any herbal remedies to your dog's diet or care routine, consult with a veterinarian. Every dog is different, and what benefits one may not be suitable for another. Your veterinarian can guide you in finding the best approach for your dog's individual health needs.

DIGESTIVE DISORDERS

Digestive issues are common in dogs and can range from mild to severe. Whether it's a bout of diarrhea after eating something they shouldn't have, chronic constipation, or ongoing nausea, these issues can significantly impact your dog's quality of life. Herbs offer gentle and effective solutions for managing these problems, supporting your dog's digestive health without harsh interventions.

Herbal Remedies for Diarrhea, Constipation, and Nausea

When your dog experiences diarrhea, it's often the body's way of expelling something harmful. However, prolonged diarrhea can lead to dehydration and nutrient loss. Slippery elm is an excellent herb for soothing the digestive tract. It works by coating the stomach and intestines with a protective layer, which helps to calm inflammation and reduce irritation. You can give slippery elm as a powder mixed with water or in capsule form to help solidify stools and reduce discomfort.

For constipation, pumpkin is a tried-and-true remedy. Rich in fiber, pumpkin helps to regulate bowel movements by adding bulk to the stool. It's gentle enough for regular use and can be added directly to your dog's food. Start with a small amount, around a teaspoon for small dogs and a tablespoon for larger breeds, and adjust as needed.

Ginger is the go-to herb for nausea. Whether your dog suffers from motion sickness or an upset stomach due to dietary indiscretion, ginger can help to calm the stomach and prevent vomiting. Fresh ginger can be grated and mixed into food, or you can use ginger tea to provide relief.

Before adding any herbal remedies to your dog's diet or care routine, be sure to consult a veterinarian. Every dog is different, and what benefits one may not be appropriate for another. Your veterinarian can provide guidance tailored to your dog's unique health needs and circumstances.

Support for Inflammatory Bowel Disease and Sensitive Stomachs

Dogs with sensitive stomachs or inflammatory bowel disease (IBD) require careful management to prevent flare-ups and maintain digestive health. Licorice root is a potent anti-inflammatory herb that soothes the lining of the gut. It's particularly beneficial for dogs with IBD, as it helps to reduce the immune system's overreaction that leads to inflammation. Licorice can be given as a tincture or a tea, making it easy to incorporate into your dog's daily routine.

Marshmallow root is another herb that works wonders for sensitive stomachs. Like slippery elm, marshmallow root creates a protective layer in the digestive tract, which helps to heal and prevent irritation. It's especially useful for dogs with acid reflux or stomach ulcers.

For overall digestive support, fennel is a gentle herb that aids in digestion and reduces gas. Fennel seeds can be ground and added to food, or you can make a fennel tea to help soothe an upset stomach.

Before adding any herbal remedies to your dog's diet or care routine, it's important to consult with a veterinarian. Every dog is different, and what benefits one may not be appropriate for another. Your veterinarian can guide you on the safest and most effective approach for your dog's individual health needs.

JOINT AND MOBILITY SUPPORT

As dogs age, joint pain and decreased mobility become common concerns. Conditions like arthritis can make it difficult for your dog to move comfortably, affecting their overall quality of life. Herbal treatments offer a natural way to manage pain and improve joint health, keeping your dog active and happy.

Managing Arthritis and Joint Pain with Anti-Inflammatory Herbs

Arthritis is a degenerative condition that causes inflammation in the joints, leading to pain and stiffness. Turmeric is one of the most effective herbs for managing arthritis in dogs. The active compound in turmeric, curcumin, has powerful anti-inflammatory properties that help to reduce swelling and pain. You can make a simple turmeric paste by mixing turmeric powder with water and a little coconut oil. Add this paste to your dog's food to help ease joint pain.

Boswellia is another herb known for its anti-inflammatory effects. Often used in Ayurvedic medicine, Boswellia helps to reduce the enzymes that contribute to inflammation, making it particularly effective for chronic joint pain. You can find Boswellia in capsule form, which makes it easy to dose according to your dog's weight.

For dogs with severe arthritis, devil's claw can provide significant relief. This herb works by blocking the pathways that produce inflammatory chemicals in the body. Devil's claw is available as a tincture or in capsules and can be given daily to help manage pain.

Before introducing any herbal remedies to your dog's diet or care routine, always consult with a veterinarian. Each dog is unique, and what works for one may not be suitable for another. Your veterinarian can help determine the best approach for your dog's specific health needs and conditions.

Herbal Recipes for Mobility Enhancement

To support your dog's mobility, you can create a homemade joint support blend using herbs like yucca, alfalfa, and ginger. Yucca helps to reduce joint inflammation, while alfalfa provides essential nutrients that support joint health. Ginger, as mentioned earlier, also has anti-inflammatory properties, making this blend a potent remedy for maintaining mobility.

Combine these herbs in equal parts, grind them into a powder, and sprinkle the mixture over your dog's food daily. This blend not only helps to manage pain but also supports overall joint function, allowing your dog to move more freely.

Before adding any herbal remedies to your dog's diet or care routine, be sure to consult a veterinarian. Every dog is different, and what benefits one may not be appropriate for another. Your veterinarian can provide guidance tailored to your dog's unique health needs and circumstances.

ANXIETY AND BEHAVIORAL ISSUES

Just like humans, dogs can suffer from anxiety and behavioral problems that impact their well-being. Whether it's separation anxiety, fear of loud noises, or hyperactivity, these issues can be challenging to manage. Herbal remedies offer a natural way to calm your dog's nerves and help them feel more secure in their environment.

Herbs to Calm Stress, Anxiety, and Hyperactivity

Valerian root is one of the most well-known herbs for calming anxiety in dogs. It works as a mild sedative, helping to reduce stress and promote relaxation without causing drowsiness. Valerian can be given as a tincture or capsule, and it's particularly useful during stressful events like thunderstorms or trips to the vet.

Lemon balm is another calming herb that can help to reduce anxiety and hyperactivity. It works by soothing the nervous system, making it easier for your dog to remain calm in situations that would normally trigger stress. You can give lemon balm as a tea or tincture, mixing it into your dog's water or food.

For dogs with chronic anxiety, passionflower can be a lifesaver. This herb helps to balance neurotransmitters in the brain, reducing anxiety and promoting a sense of well-being. Passionflower is safe for long-term use and can be given daily to help manage anxiety.

Before adding any herbal remedies to your dog's diet or care routine, consult with a veterinarian. Every dog is different, and what benefits one may not be suitable for another. Your veterinarian can guide you in finding the best approach for your dog's individual health needs.

Using Herbal Support for Separation Anxiety and Travel

Separation anxiety is a common issue for many dogs, particularly those who are very attached to their owners. Skullcap is an herb that can help ease the symptoms of separation anxiety by calming the nervous system and reducing stress. Skullcap can be used alongside other calming herbs like valerian or passionflower for a more comprehensive approach to managing anxiety.

When traveling with your dog, ginger can help to prevent motion sickness and calm nerves. As mentioned earlier, ginger is great for nausea, but it also has calming properties that can make travel less stressful for your dog. Give your dog a small piece of fresh ginger or a ginger capsule about 30 minutes before travel to help prevent motion sickness.

Chamomile is another excellent herb for travel anxiety. Its gentle sedative effects help to relax your dog without making them too sleepy. You can give chamomile as a tea or tincture before traveling to help your dog feel more at ease.

Before adding any herbal remedies to your dog's diet or care routine, be sure to consult a veterinarian. Every dog is different, and what benefits one may not be appropriate for another. Your veterinarian can provide guidance tailored to your dog's unique health needs and circumstances.

IMMUNE SYSTEM SUPPORT

A strong immune system is crucial for your dog's overall health, helping to ward off infections and chronic diseases. Herbs can play a significant role in boosting your dog's immune system, providing them with the resilience they need to stay healthy.

Strengthening the Immune System with Herbs

Echinacea is one of the most popular herbs for immune support. It helps to stimulate the production of white blood cells, which are essential for fighting off infections. You can give echinacea as a tincture or in capsule form, particularly during times when your dog's immune system might be compromised, such as after surgery or during illness.

Astragalus is another powerful immune-boosting herb. It works by enhancing the body's resistance to stress and disease, making it a great herb for long-term immune support. Astragalus can be added to your dog's food as a powder or given as a tincture.

For dogs prone to infections, olive leaf is a potent antimicrobial herb that can help to prevent and treat infections. Olive leaf extract can be given daily to support your dog's immune system and protect against pathogens.

Before adding any herbal remedies to your dog's diet or care routine, it's important to consult with a veterinarian. Every dog is different, and what benefits one may not be appropriate for another. Your veterinarian can guide you on the safest and most effective approach for your dog's individual health needs.

Remedies for Chronic Infections and Autoimmune Issues

Chronic infections can be tough to manage, especially if your dog has an underlying autoimmune condition. Goldenseal is a powerful herb with antimicrobial and anti-inflammatory properties, making it effective for treating chronic infections. It's particularly useful for infections of the respiratory tract, digestive system, and skin. Goldenseal is best given as a tincture, and it's important to use it in cycles (e.g., two weeks on, one week off) to avoid potential side effects.

Astragalus is, again, a valuable herb for autoimmune issues. It helps to regulate the immune system, making it less likely to overreact and attack the body's own tissues. This makes astragalus especially useful for dogs with conditions like lupus or autoimmune thyroiditis.

Reishi mushroom is another excellent herb for managing autoimmune conditions. Reishi helps to balance the immune system and reduce inflammation, which is critical for managing autoimmune diseases. You can give reishi as a powder mixed into food or as a supplement.

Before introducing any herbal remedies to your dog's diet or care routine, always consult with a veterinarian. Each dog is unique, and what works for one may not be suitable for another. Your veterinarian can help determine the best approach for your dog's specific health needs and conditions.

LIVER AND KIDNEY HEALTH

The liver and kidneys are vital organs that play a crucial role in detoxification and overall health. Supporting these organs with herbs can help to improve your dog's ability to eliminate toxins and maintain optimal health.

Detoxifying the Liver with Milk Thistle and Dandelion

Milk thistle is the go-to herb for liver health. It contains silymarin, a compound that helps to regenerate liver cells and protect the liver from damage. Milk thistle can be given as a tincture or in capsule form, particularly if your dog has been exposed to toxins or is on long-term medication.

Dandelion is another excellent herb for liver detoxification. It stimulates bile production, which aids in digestion and helps the liver eliminate toxins more effectively. You can give dandelion as a tea or tincture or add fresh dandelion greens to your dog's food.

Before adding any herbal remedies to your dog's diet or care routine, consult with a veterinarian. Every dog is different, and what benefits one may not be suitable for another. Your veterinarian can guide you in finding the best approach for your dog's individual health needs.

Supporting Renal Function with Herbs for Kidney Health

For kidney health, nettles are an excellent choice. Nettles are a natural diuretic, helping to flush out toxins and reduce inflammation in the kidneys. You can give nettles as tea or in capsule form to support kidney function.

Cranberry is well-known for its ability to prevent urinary tract infections, but it also supports overall kidney health. Cranberry helps to prevent bacteria from adhering to the urinary tract, reducing the risk of infection. You can give cranberry as a powder mixed into food or as a supplement.

Horsetail is another herb that supports kidney health. It's rich in silica, which helps to strengthen connective tissue and reduce inflammation in the kidneys. Horsetail can be given as tea or in capsule form to support renal function. Before adding any herbal remedies to your dog's diet or care routine, be sure to consult a veterinarian. Every dog is different, and what benefits one may not be appropriate for another. Your veterinarian can provide guidance tailored to your dog's unique health needs and circumstances.

CARDIOVASCULAR AND RESPIRATORY HEALTH

Keeping your dog's heart and lungs healthy is essential for their overall well-being. Herbs can provide natural support for cardiovascular and respiratory health, helping to manage conditions like heart disease and respiratory infections.

Herbal Support for Heart Health

Hawthorn is one of the best herbs for heart health. It strengthens the heart muscle, improves circulation, and helps to regulate blood pressure. Hawthorn can be given as a tincture or in capsule form, making it easy to incorporate into your dog's daily routine.

Motherwort is another herb that supports heart health by reducing anxiety and promoting relaxation. This can be particularly beneficial for dogs with heart conditions that are exacerbated by stress. Motherwort can be given as a tincture or mixed into food. Garlic is known for its cardiovascular benefits, particularly its ability to lower cholesterol and improve circulation. While garlic should be used in moderation, a small amount can be beneficial for heart health. You can add fresh, finely minced garlic to your dog's food, starting with a small amount and gradually increasing it. Before adding any herbal remedies to your dog's diet or care routine, it's important to consult with a veterinarian. Every dog is different, and what benefits one may not be appropriate for another. Your veterinarian can guide you on the safest and most effective approach for your dog's individual health needs.

Managing Respiratory Issues with Natural Remedies

Respiratory issues like kennel cough or bronchitis can be distressing for your dog. Thyme is an excellent herb for respiratory health, as it has antibacterial and expectorant properties. Thyme can be given as a tea or tincture to help clear mucus and reduce coughing.

Licorice root is another herb that supports respiratory health by soothing the mucous membranes and reducing inflammation. It's particularly useful for dogs with chronic respiratory conditions. Licorice can be given as a tincture or in capsule form. For dogs with chronic respiratory issues, mullein is a gentle herb that helps to clear the lungs and improve breathing. Mullein can be given as a tea or tincture, and it's safe for long-term use.

Before introducing any herbal remedies to your dog's diet or care routine, always consult with a veterinarian. Each dog is unique, and what works for one may not be suitable for another. Your veterinarian can help determine the best approach for your dog's specific health needs and conditions.

THE BOTTOM LINE

In this chapter, you've explored how to address some of the most common health issues in dogs using herbal treatments. From skin and coat problems to digestive disorders, joint pain, and anxiety, you've learned about the power of natural remedies. Herbs like turmeric, chamomile, and milk thistle can provide real relief and support for your dog's overall well-being. By understanding the symptoms and applying these treatments, you're not just treating the issue—you're boosting your dog's health in a gentle, effective way.

Now that you've got a solid grasp of how herbs can support specific ailments, it's time to get even more hands-on. In the next chapter, you'll find step-by-step instructions for creating remedies that you can start using right away. Whether it's a soothing balm for irritated skin or a calming tea for anxiety, you're about to discover how to make these natural solutions at home. Let's dive into some practical recipes that will take your dog's care to the next level!

BONUS EXTRA!!!

Scan the QR CODE and GET Your Bonuses:

1. ESSENTIAL CANINE FIRST AID
2. GROWING YOUR OWN MEDICINAL HERB GARDEN
3. EASY HOMEMADE DOG TREAT RECIPES
4. A-Z GUIDE OF HERBS SAFE FOR DOGS

As SPAM Filters Are Pretty Crazy These Days...
...WHITELIST this Email Address!

info@floraandwaterpublishing.com

In This Way, Your Bonus Will Appear in the Main Folder of Your INBOX and They Will Not Be Buried Along With Other Advertisements in Your PROMOTION/SPAM Folder.

HERE IS HOW TO DO IT:
From Android Smartphone/Tablet
Open the Contacts App;
In the lower right corner, tap + (Add);
Enter the name and email address and then tap Save.

From iPhone/iPad
Open the Contacts App;
In the upper right corner, tap + (Add);
Enter the name and email address and then tap Finish.

Thank You for Your Support!

Your support means so much, and I hope 'The Canine Herbal Remedies Bible' has empowered you to care for your dog's health naturally and confidently.

If you found this guide helpful, would you consider sharing your experience in a review on Amazon?

Your feedback helps others discover safe, natural ways to care for their pets—and it allows me to continue creating resources to support you and your furry friend!

Simply scan the QR code below to leave your review.

Thank you for being part of this journey toward healthier, happier dogs!

Real-Life Natural Remedy Recipes

CHAPTER 5

"When crafting natural remedy recipes, it's important to remember that each component should serve a purpose in restoring balance, whether you're treating a cold, soothing skin irritation, or boosting immunity." – James A. Duke

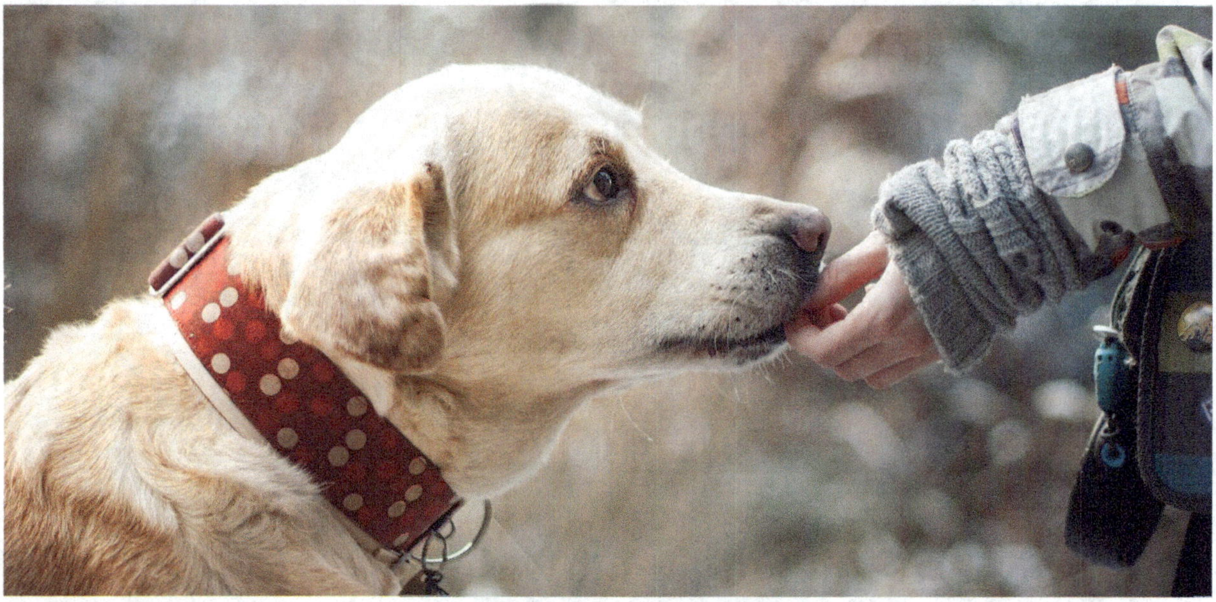

Taking care of your dog's health naturally can feel empowering. There's a special kind of joy in knowing that you can create something at home that will keep your furry friend happy and healthy. The good news? Making your own herbal remedies doesn't have to be complicated. Whether you're interested in supporting your dog's immune system, calming them during stressful situations, or helping their joints stay strong and limber, this chapter will guide you step by step. By the end, you'll have a variety of practical recipes that you can whip up right in your kitchen, using simple ingredients you likely already have.

Let's dive into everyday health recipes that will keep your dog thriving, from digestion support to detoxification. These DIY remedies are safe and easy to make, so even if you're new to herbal medicine, you'll feel confident preparing them. Your dog deserves the best care, and with these recipes, you'll be able to give them just that.

EVERYDAY HEALTH RECIPES

Everyday health maintenance is essential for your dog's long-term well-being. Simple herbal remedies can support your dog's overall health, helping with common issues like anxiety, digestion, skin irritations, and joint discomfort. By incorporating gentle, natural ingredients into their routine, you can promote balance and vitality. This section provides easy-to-make herbal blends, each tailored to address specific health concerns, ensuring your dog stays happy and healthy. Remember to always consult your vet before introducing new remedies into your dog's diet.

Simple Herbal Blends for General Wellness

Herbal remedies can be a great way to naturally support your dog's overall health and well-being. These simple blends harness the power of herbs to address common issues like anxiety, skin irritation, digestion, and joint health. By using calming, immune-boosting, and anti-inflammatory herbs, you can create gentle, natural solutions to keep your dog healthy. Always consult your vet before introducing new herbs into your dog's routine to ensure they're safe and effective for your dog's specific needs.

Calming Chamomile & Lavender Blend

This blend helps reduce anxiety and promotes relaxation in dogs. Chamomile and lavender are known for their calming properties, making this ideal for stressed or anxious dogs.

Ingredients:
- 1 tablespoon dried chamomile flowers
- 1 teaspoon dried lavender flowers
- 1 teaspoon dried lemon balm
- 1 cup water

Instructions:
- Boil the water and remove it from the heat.
- Add the chamomile, lavender, and lemon balm to the water.
- Let it steep for 10 minutes.
- Strain the liquid to remove the herbs.
- Allow the blend to cool completely before use.

Dosing Guidelines:
- Small dogs: 1 teaspoon, twice a day.
- Medium dogs: 1 tablespoon, twice a day.
- Large dogs: 2 tablespoons, twice a day.

Tips for Storage:
Store in a sealed container in the refrigerator for up to 3 days. Discard if it changes color or develops a sour smell.

Immune Boosting Echinacea & Astragalus Blend

This blend strengthens your dog's immune system and supports overall health. Echinacea and astragalus are both known for their immune-boosting properties.

Ingredients:
- 1 tablespoon dried echinacea root
- 1 teaspoon dried astragalus root
- 1 cup water

Instructions:
- Add echinacea and astragalus to a pot with water.
- Bring to a boil and then simmer for 15 minutes.
- Strain the liquid and let it cool.
- Store in a glass bottle or jar.

Dosing Guidelines:
- Small dogs: 1/2 teaspoon, once a day.
- Medium dogs: 1 teaspoon, once a day.
- Large dogs: 1 tablespoon, once a day.

Tips for Storage:
Keep in an airtight container in the refrigerator for up to 5 days.

Skin Soothing Calendula e Nettle Blend

This blend soothes irritated skin and promotes healing. Calendula is excellent for skin repair, and nettle helps reduce inflammation.

Ingredients:

- 1 tablespoon dried calendula flowers
- 1 teaspoon dried nettle leaves
- 1 cup water

Instructions:

- Heat water until boiling, then remove from heat.
- Add calendula and nettle to the water.
- Steep for 15 minutes, then strain.
- Let the liquid cool before applying it to your dog's skin.

Dosing Guidelines:

- Apply externally to affected areas using a clean cloth.
- For internal use: Small dogs: 1 teaspoon, Medium dogs: 1 tablespoon, Large dogs: 2 tablespoons (once a day).

Tips for Storage:

Store in the fridge for up to 3 days and use fresh applications as needed.

Digestive Aid Ginger e Fennel Blend

This herbal blend supports digestion and helps with bloating and gas. Ginger soothes the stomach, while fennel improves digestion.

Ingredients:

- 1 teaspoon dried ginger root
- 1 teaspoon fennel seeds
- 1 cup water

Instructions:

- Boil the water, then add ginger and fennel seeds.
- Simmer for 10 minutes and then strain.
- Allow it to cool before giving it to your dog.

Dosing Guidelines:

- Small dogs: 1/4 teaspoon, twice a day.
- Medium dogs: 1/2 teaspoon, twice a day.
- Large dogs: 1 teaspoon, twice a day.

Tips for Storage:

Store in an airtight container in the fridge for up to 3 days.

Joint Health Turmeric e Burdock Root Blend

This blend promotes joint health and reduces inflammation. Turmeric is known for its anti-inflammatory properties, and burdock root helps detoxify and support mobility.

Ingredients:
- 1 teaspoon ground turmeric
- 1 teaspoon dried burdock root
- 1 cup water

Instructions:
- Boil the water and add turmeric and burdock root.
- Let it simmer for 15 minutes, stirring occasionally.
- Strain the liquid and let it cool.

Dosing Guidelines:
- Small dogs: 1/4 teaspoon, once a day.
- Medium dogs: 1/2 teaspoon, once a day.
- Large dogs: 1 teaspoon, once a day.

Tips for Storage:
Store in the fridge for up to 5 days. Shake well before use. These recipes offer a natural way to support your dog's wellness through herbal remedies. Make sure to consult your vet before adding new herbs to your dog's routine.

Recipes for Boosting Immune Function

Supporting your dog's immune system with natural herbal remedies is a gentle yet effective way to promote overall health. Herbs such as elderberry, echinacea, turmeric, and astragalus are known for their immune-boosting properties and can be incorporated into your dog's diet in various forms. The following recipes provide simple, safe ways to enhance your dog's natural defenses. As always, consult your veterinarian before adding new herbs to your dog's routine, especially if they have underlying health conditions.

Elderberry e Echinacea Immune Booster

This herbal blend combines elderberry and echinacea, both of which are known for their immune-boosting properties, to support your dog's natural defenses.

Ingredients:
- 1 tablespoon dried elderberries
- 1 teaspoon dried echinacea root
- 1 cup water

Instructions:
- Bring the water to a boil.
- Add elderberries and echinacea root to the boiling water.
- Reduce heat and simmer for 10 minutes.
- Strain the liquid and allow it to cool completely.

Dosing Guidelines:
- Small dogs: 1/4 teaspoon, twice a day.
- Medium dogs: 1/2 teaspoon, twice a day.
- Large dogs: 1 teaspoon, twice a day.

Tips for Storage:
Store in the refrigerator for up to 4 days. Discard if the liquid changes color or develops an unusual smell.

Turmeric & Coconut Oil Golden Paste

This immune-boosting paste features turmeric, which has powerful anti-inflammatory properties, and coconut oil, known for its immune-enhancing benefits.

Ingredients:

- 1/4 cup turmeric powder
- 1/2 cup water
- 1/4 cup coconut oil
- 1/2 teaspoon ground black pepper (to enhance absorption)

Instructions:

- Mix the turmeric powder and water in a saucepan.
- Heat on low, stirring constantly, until it forms a paste (about 7-10 minutes).
- Remove from heat and add the coconut oil and black pepper, stirring to combine.
- Let it cool before use.

Dosing Guidelines:

- Small dogs: 1/4 teaspoon, once a day.
- Medium dogs: 1/2 teaspoon, once a day.
- Large dogs: 1 teaspoon, once a day.

Tips for Storage:

Store in an airtight container in the refrigerator for up to 2 weeks. Stir before each use.

Astragalus & Mushroom Immune Support Blend

Astragalus and medicinal mushrooms like reishi and shiitake boost immune function by stimulating your dog's natural defense mechanisms.

Ingredients:

- 1 teaspoon dried astragalus root
- 1 teaspoon dried reishi mushroom
- 1 teaspoon dried shiitake mushroom
- 1 cup water

Instructions:

- Bring the water to a boil, then reduce to a simmer.
- Add astragalus, reishi, and shiitake mushrooms to the water.
- Simmer for 20 minutes, then strain the liquid.
- Let it cool completely before serving.

Dosing Guidelines:

- Small dogs: 1/2 teaspoon, once a day.
- Medium dogs: 1 teaspoon, once a day.
- Large dogs: 1 tablespoon, once a day.

Tips for Storage:

Keep refrigerated for up to 3 days in a sealed container.

Garlic & Thyme Immune Tonic

Garlic and thyme are both rich in antioxidants and help enhance immune function. This blend is ideal for dogs needing extra immune support.

Ingredients:
- 1 clove garlic, finely chopped (adjust for small dogs)
- 1 teaspoon dried thyme
- 1 cup water

Instructions:
- Boil the water and add the thyme and garlic.
- Reduce to a simmer and let it cook for 10 minutes.
- Strain and cool before use.

Dosing Guidelines:
- Small dogs: 1/4 teaspoon, once a day.
- Medium dogs: 1/2 teaspoon, once a day.
- Large dogs: 1 teaspoon, once a day.

Tips for Storage:
Store in the refrigerator for up to 3 days in an airtight container.

Rosehip & Nettle Vitamin C Booster

Rosehips are rich in Vitamin C, an essential nutrient for immune health. Nettle adds anti-inflammatory and antioxidant properties to support overall wellness.

Ingredients:
- 1 tablespoon dried rosehips
- 1 teaspoon dried nettle leaves
- 1 cup water

Instructions:
- Bring the water to a boil.
- Add rosehips and nettle leaves.
- Reduce the heat and simmer for 10 minutes.
- Strain the liquid and let it cool before serving.

Dosing Guidelines:
- Small dogs: 1/4 teaspoon, twice a day.
- Medium dogs: 1/2 teaspoon, twice a day.
- Large dogs: 1 teaspoon, twice a day.

Tips for Storage:
Store in an airtight container in the refrigerator for up to 5 days.
These recipes offer natural ways to enhance your dog's immune system. Be sure to consult with a veterinarian before introducing new herbs into your dog's diet.

DIGESTIVE HEALTH RECIPES

Digestive health is crucial for your dog's overall well-being. A smooth-running digestive system ensures your dog absorbs essential nutrients while minimizing discomfort, bloating, or gas. Herbal teas and powders can offer natural support, using ingredients like chamomile, ginger, and slippery elm to soothe your dog's stomach. This section provides easy-to-prepare remedies that help alleviate common digestive issues while promoting gut health. As always, consult your vet before adding any new herbs to your dog's routine.

Herbal Teas and Powders for Digestive Comfort

Herbal teas and powders can be a gentle, natural way to support your dog's digestive health. Many herbs possess properties that help alleviate common issues like bloating, gas, nausea, and constipation. Chamomile, ginger, and slippery elm are just a few examples of herbs that can soothe the digestive tract and reduce inflammation. In this section, you'll learn how to prepare simple yet effective herbal remedies that offer comfort to your dog's stomach while promoting overall gut health.

Chamomile e Fennel Digestive Tea

This soothing herbal tea helps relieve gas, bloating, and digestive discomfort in dogs. Chamomile calms the stomach, while fennel aids digestion.

Ingredients:
- 1 teaspoon dried chamomile flowers
- 1/2 teaspoon fennel seeds
- 1 cup water

Instructions:
- Boil the water, then remove from heat.
- Add chamomile and fennel seeds to the water.
- Let it steep for 10 minutes.
- Strain the tea and allow it to cool completely before offering it to your dog.

Dosing Guidelines:
- Small dogs: 1-2 teaspoons, twice a day.
- Medium dogs: 1 tablespoon, twice a day.
- Large dogs: 2 tablespoons, twice a day.

Tips for Storage:

Store in the refrigerator for up to 2 days. Discard if it develops a sour smell.

Ginger e Peppermint Tummy Soother Tea

This tea helps settle upset stomachs, relieve nausea, and reduce gas. Ginger and peppermint are well-known for their digestive benefits.

Ingredients:

- 1/2 teaspoon dried ginger root
- 1/2 teaspoon dried peppermint leaves
- 1 cup water

Instructions:

- Boil the water and remove it from the heat.
- Add ginger and peppermint to the water.
- Steep for 10 minutes and strain the tea.
- Let it cool before serving.

Dosing Guidelines:

- Small dogs: 1 teaspoon, twice a day.
- Medium dogs: 1 tablespoon, twice a day.
- Large dogs: 2 tablespoons, twice a day.

Tips for Storage:

Keep in a sealed container in the fridge for up to 3 days.

Slippery Elm e Licorice Root Digestive Aid Tea

Slippery elm coats the digestive tract, reducing inflammation and soothing discomfort, while licorice root enhances the blend's digestive benefits.

Ingredients:

- 1 teaspoon slippery elm powder
- 1/2 teaspoon dried licorice root
- 1 cup water

Instructions:

- Bring water to a boil, then remove from heat.
- Add the slippery elm powder and licorice root to the water.
- Stir well and steep for 5 minutes.
- Strain the tea and allow it to cool.

Dosing Guidelines:

- Small dogs: 1 teaspoon, twice a day.
- Medium dogs: 1 tablespoon, twice a day.
- Large dogs: 2 tablespoons, twice a day.

Tips for Storage:

Store in the refrigerator for up to 3 days. Shake well before use.

Pumpkin & Ginger Digestive Powder

This digestive powder helps relieve constipation and soothe an upset stomach. Pumpkin is rich in fiber, while ginger calms digestive discomfort.

Ingredients:
- 1 tablespoon dried pumpkin powder
- 1/2 teaspoon ground ginger

Instructions:
- Mix the dried pumpkin powder and ground ginger in a bowl.
- Store in an airtight container.

Dosing Guidelines:
- Small dogs: 1/4 teaspoon, mixed into food.
- Medium dogs: 1/2 teaspoon, mixed into food.
- Large dogs: 1 teaspoon, mixed into food.

Tips for Storage:
Store in a cool, dry place for up to 6 months.

Turmeric & Fennel Digestive Powder

This anti-inflammatory blend of turmeric and fennel helps improve digestion and reduces gas in dogs. It also supports liver function.

Ingredients:
- 1 tablespoon ground turmeric
- 1/2 teaspoon ground fennel seeds

Instructions:
- Combine the ground turmeric and fennel in a bowl.
- Mix thoroughly and store in a sealed jar.

Dosing Guidelines:
- Small dogs: 1/8 teaspoon, mixed into food.
- Medium dogs: 1/4 teaspoon, mixed into food.
- Large dogs: 1/2 teaspoon, mixed into food.

Tips for Storage:
Store in a cool, dry place for up to 6 months.

Slippery Elm & Marshmallow Root Digestive Powder

This powder helps soothe the digestive tract, reduce inflammation, and support overall gut health. Slippery elm and marshmallow roots create a protective coating.

Ingredients:

- 1 tablespoon slippery elm powder
- 1/2 teaspoon marshmallow root powder

Instructions:

- Mix the slippery elm and marshmallow root powders in a bowl.
- Store in a tightly sealed container.

Dosing Guidelines:

- Small dogs: 1/4 teaspoon, mixed with water or food.
- Medium dogs: 1/2 teaspoon, mixed with water or food.
- Large dogs: 1 teaspoon, mixed with water or food.

Tips for Storage:

Keep in a dry place, sealed, for up to 6 months. These herbal teas and powders provide natural digestive relief for dogs, helping to ease discomfort and promote overall gut health. Be sure to consult your vet before introducing new herbs into your dog's diet.

Healing Bone Broth with Medicinal Herbs

Bone broths infused with medicinal herbs provide a wealth of nutrients and healing benefits for dogs, supporting joint health, digestion, immune function, and overall wellness. The combination of marrow-rich bones with powerful anti-inflammatory, detoxifying, and soothing herbs makes these broths an excellent addition to your dog's diet. Whether your goal is to alleviate joint pain, boost immunity, or promote calmness, these healing broths are a natural and effective solution. Always consult your vet before introducing new ingredients to your dog's diet

Turmeric & Ginger Bone Broth

This healing bone broth combines the anti-inflammatory properties of turmeric and ginger with the nutritional benefits of bone broth to promote joint health and overall wellness in dogs.

Ingredients:

- 2 pounds of beef or chicken bones (with marrow)
- 1 tablespoon ground turmeric
- 1 teaspoon grated fresh ginger
- 10 cups water
- 1 tablespoon apple cider vinegar

Dosing Guidelines:

- Small dogs: 1-2 tablespoons, once a day.
- Medium dogs: 1/4 cup, once a day.
- Large dogs: 1/2 cup, once a day.

Tips for Storage:

Store in the refrigerator for up to 5 days or freeze in portions for up to 3 months.

Instructions:

1. Place the bones in a large pot and cover them with water.
2. Add apple cider vinegar to help extract nutrients from the bones.
3. Bring the mixture to a boil, then reduce the heat to a simmer.
4. Add the turmeric and ginger.
5. Simmer the broth for 12-24 hours, skimming off any foam.
6. Strain the broth and let it cool.

Parsley e Nettle Bone Broth

Parsley and nettle are both rich in vitamins and minerals, making this broth a great option for boosting your dog's immune system and promoting healthy digestion.

Ingredients:
- 2 pounds of chicken or beef bones
- 1 tablespoon dried nettle leaves
- 1 tablespoon fresh parsley, chopped
- 10 cups water
- 1 tablespoon apple cider vinegar

Instructions:
- Place the bones in a large pot and cover them with water.
- Add apple cider vinegar and bring the mixture to a boil.
- Lower the heat to a simmer, add nettle and parsley, and cook for 12-24 hours.
- Strain the broth and allow it to cool.

Dosing Guidelines:
- Small dogs: 2 tablespoons, once a day.
- Medium dogs: 1/4 cup, once a day.
- Large dogs: 1/2 cup, once a day.

Tips for Storage:
Store in the fridge for up to 5 days or freeze in portions for up to 3 months.

Chamomile e Lavender Bone Broth

This calming bone broth, infused with chamomile and lavender, helps soothe anxiety and digestive issues while providing the nutritional benefits of bone broth.

Ingredients:
- 2 pounds of beef bones
- 1 tablespoon dried chamomile flowers
- 1 teaspoon dried lavender flowers
- 10 cups water
- 1 tablespoon apple cider vinegar

Instructions:
- Add bones to a pot, cover with water, and add apple cider vinegar.
- Bring to a boil, then simmer.
- Add chamomile and lavender to the pot and simmer for 12-24 hours.
- Strain the broth and let it cool before serving.

Dosing Guidelines:
- Small dogs: 1-2 tablespoons, twice a day.
- Medium dogs: 1/4 cup, twice a day.
- Large dogs: 1/2 cup, twice a day.

Tips for Storage:
Store in the refrigerator for up to 4 days or freeze in portions for up to 3 months.

Dandelion e Burdock Root Bone Broth

Dandelion and burdock root are excellent for supporting liver health and detoxification. This bone broth combines these herbs with the healing properties of marrow bones for overall wellness.

Ingredients:
- 2 pounds of beef or lamb bones
- 1 tablespoon dried dandelion root
- 1 tablespoon dried burdock root
- 10 cups water
- 1 tablespoon apple cider vinegar

Instructions:
- Place bones in a pot, cover with water, and add apple cider vinegar.
- Bring the mixture to a boil and then lower to a simmer.
- Add dandelion and burdock root to the broth.
- Simmer for 12-24 hours, then strain the broth.

Dosing Guidelines:
- Small dogs: 2 tablespoons, once a day.
- Medium dogs: 1/4 cup, once a day.
- Large dogs: 1/2 cup, once a day.

Tips for Storage:
Store in the refrigerator for 4-5 days or freeze for up to 3 months.

Rosemary e Thyme Bone Broth

Rosemary and thyme are natural antioxidants and anti-inflammatory herbs that support your dog's digestive and immune systems. Combined with bone broth, this recipe aids in overall wellness.

Ingredients:
- 2 pounds of chicken bones
- 1 teaspoon dried rosemary
- 1 teaspoon dried thyme
- 10 cups water
- 1 tablespoon apple cider vinegar

Instructions:
- Add bones, water, and apple cider vinegar to a pot and bring to a boil.
- Lower the heat to a simmer and add rosemary and thyme.
- Simmer for 12-24 hours, skimming any foam that forms on top.
- Strain and let the broth cool before serving.

Dosing Guidelines:
- Small dogs: 1-2 tablespoons, twice a day.
- Medium dogs: 1/4 cup, twice a day.
- Large dogs: 1/2 cup, twice a day.

Tips for Storage:
Store in the refrigerator for up to 5 days or freeze in individual portions for up to 3 months.
These bone broths offer a nourishing and healing boost for your dog's overall health.
Always consult with a vet before adding new herbs to your dog's diet.

CALMING REMEDIES

Dogs often experience anxiety due to triggers like thunderstorms or being left alone. Using natural calming remedies can offer gentle, non-pharmaceutical solutions to ease their stress. Herbal relaxation treats, made with calming ingredients like chamomile, lavender, valerian root, and lemon balm, provide a simple yet effective way to reduce anxiety. These homemade recipes are easy to prepare and safe for your dog. Always consult your vet before introducing new herbs to ensure they suit your dog's specific needs.

Herbal Relaxation Treats

Herbal treats can be a simple and effective way to help your dog relax and reduce anxiety. Ingredients like chamomile, lavender, valerian root, and lemon balm are known for their calming effects and can be safely incorporated into homemade dog treats. These recipes are easy to make, using common ingredients and herbs that are gentle on your dog's system. Always check with your veterinarian before introducing new herbs to ensure they are safe for your dog's specific health needs.

Chamomile e Lavender Relaxation Biscuits

These calming biscuits are infused with chamomile and lavender, both known for their ability to promote relaxation and reduce anxiety in dogs.

Ingredients:

- 1 cup whole wheat flour
- 1/2 cup rolled oats
- 1 tablespoon dried chamomile flowers
- 1 teaspoon dried lavender flowers
- 1/4 cup unsweetened applesauce
- 1 egg
- 1/4 cup water

Instructions:

- Preheat the oven to 350°F (175°C).
- In a large bowl, mix the flour, oats, chamomile, and lavender.
- In a separate bowl, whisk the egg and applesauce.
- Gradually combine the wet ingredients with the dry ingredients.
- Add water as needed to form a dough.
- Roll out the dough and cut it into biscuit shapes.
- Place the biscuits on a baking sheet and bake for 20 minutes or until golden brown.
- Let them cool completely before serving.

Dosing Guidelines:

- Small dogs: 1 biscuit, once a day.
- Medium dogs: 2 biscuits, once a day.
- Large dogs: 3 biscuits, once a day.

Tips for Storage:

Store in an airtight container at room temperature for up to a week, or refrigerate for up to 2 weeks.

Valerian & Honey Calming Bites

Valerian root is known for its soothing effects on anxiety, while honey adds a touch of sweetness and promotes relaxation.

Ingredients:
- 1 cup brown rice flour
- 1 teaspoon dried valerian root powder
- 2 tablespoons raw honey
- 1/4 cup peanut butter (unsweetened)
- 1/2 cup water

Instructions:
- Preheat the oven to 325°F (160°C).
- In a bowl, mix brown rice flour and valerian root powder.
- Add the honey and peanut butter, then gradually mix in the water to form a dough.
- Roll the dough into small bite-sized balls and place them on a baking sheet.
- Bake for 15-20 minutes until firm.
- Let them cool completely before serving.

Dosing Guidelines:
- Small dogs: 1 bite, once a day.
- Medium dogs: 2 bites, once a day.
- Large dogs: 3 bites, once a day.

Tips for Storage:
Store in the fridge for up to 2 weeks or freeze for up to 3 months.

Lemon Balm & Coconut Oil Relaxation Treats

Lemon balm helps reduce stress and anxiety, while coconut oil promotes overall wellness. These treats are easy to make and packed with calming benefits.

Ingredients:
- 1/2 cup coconut oil (melted)
- 1 tablespoon dried lemon balm
- 1/4 cup unsweetened pumpkin puree
- 1/2 cup oat flour

Instructions:
- Preheat the oven to 350°F (175°C).
- In a bowl, mix the coconut oil, lemon balm, and pumpkin puree.
- Gradually add the oat flour until a dough forms.
- Roll the dough into small balls and place them on a baking sheet.
- Bake for 15-18 minutes until firm.
- Let the treats cool completely before serving.

Dosing Guidelines:
- Small dogs: 1 treat, once a day.
- Medium dogs: 2 treats, once a day.
- Large dogs: 3 treats, once a day.

Tips for Storage:
- Store in an airtight container in the fridge for up to 2 weeks.

Passionflower e Peanut Butter Dog Treats

Passionflower is great for reducing anxiety and promoting calmness in dogs. Combined with peanut butter, this makes a delicious and soothing treat.

Ingredients:

- 1 cup whole wheat flour
- 1 teaspoon dried passionflower powder
- 1/2 cup unsweetened peanut butter
- 1/4 cup water
- 1 egg

Instructions:

- Preheat the oven to 350°F (175°C).
- In a bowl, mix the flour and passionflower powder.
- Add the peanut butter, egg, and water, stirring until a dough forms.
- Roll out the dough and cut it into small shapes.
- Place the shapes on a baking sheet and bake for 20 minutes or until golden brown.
- Let them cool completely before serving.

Dosing Guidelines:

- Small dogs: 1 treat, once a day.
- Medium dogs: 2 treats, once a day.
- Large dogs: 3 treats, once a day.

Tips for Storage:

Store in an airtight container at room temperature for up to a week or refrigerate for up to 2 weeks.

Oat e Chamomile Calming Cookies

Oats and chamomile are perfect for calming your dog's nerves. These cookies are gentle on the stomach and great for relaxation.

Ingredients:

- 1 cup rolled oats (ground into flour)
- 1 tablespoon dried chamomile flowers
- 1/4 cup applesauce
- 1/4 cup peanut butter (unsweetened)
- 1/4 cup water

Instructions:

- Preheat the oven to 350°F (175°C).
- In a large bowl, mix the oat flour and chamomile.
- Add applesauce, peanut butter, and water, stirring until a dough forms.
- Roll the dough into small cookies and place them on a baking sheet.
- Bake for 15-20 minutes until firm.
- Let them cool before serving.

Dosing Guidelines:

- Small dogs: 1 cookie, once a day.
- Medium dogs: 2 cookies, once a day.
- Large dogs: 3 cookies, once a day.

Tips for Storage:

Store in a sealed container at room temperature for up to a week or refrigerate for 2 weeks. These herbal relaxation treats offer natural, safe ways to help calm and soothe your dog. Always consult your vet before introducing new herbs to your dog's diet.

Anxiety-Reducing Teas and Tonics

Herbal teas and tonics can be a wonderful, natural solution to help calm your dog's anxiety and stress. Herbs like chamomile, lavender, valerian root, and ashwagandha are well-known for their calming and relaxing properties, making them effective for dogs prone to anxiety. These recipes are simple to prepare and safe when used in moderation. Always consult your veterinarian before introducing new herbs to ensure they are appropriate for your dog's specific health needs.

Chamomile e Lemon Balm Soothing Tea

This calming tea helps reduce anxiety and promotes relaxation in dogs. Chamomile and lemon balm are known for their gentle sedative properties.

Ingredients:

- 1 teaspoon dried chamomile flowers
- 1/2 teaspoon dried lemon balm
- 1 cup water

Instructions:

- Boil the water and remove it from the heat.
- Add chamomile and lemon balm to the hot water.
- Let it steep for 10 minutes, then strain the herbs.
- Allow the tea to cool completely before offering it to your dog.

Dosing Guidelines:

- Small dogs: 1 teaspoon, twice a day.
- Medium dogs: 1 tablespoon, twice a day.
- Large dogs: 2 tablespoons, twice a day.

Tips for Storage:

Store in the refrigerator for up to 3 days. Discard if it changes color or develops a sour smell.

Lavender e Valerian Root Relaxation Tea

Lavender and valerian root are powerful herbs for calming the nervous system, making this tea an excellent choice for anxious dogs.

Ingredients:

- 1 teaspoon dried lavender flowers
- 1/2 teaspoon dried valerian root
- 1 cup water

Instructions:

- Boil the water and remove it from the heat.
- Add lavender and valerian root to the water.
- Steep for 10 minutes, then strain the liquid.
- Let it cool before giving it to your dog.

Dosing Guidelines:

- Small dogs: 1 teaspoon, once a day.
- Medium dogs: 1 tablespoon, once a day.
- Large dogs: 2 tablespoons, once a day.

Tips for Storage:

Store in a sealed container in the refrigerator for up to 3 days.

Passionflower e Peppermint Calm Tea

This tea combines passionflower, known for reducing anxiety, with peppermint, which soothes digestive discomfort often linked to stress.

Ingredients:

- 1/2 teaspoon dried passionflower
- 1/2 teaspoon dried peppermint leaves
- 1 cup water

Instructions:

- Boil the water and remove it from the heat.
- Add the passionflower and peppermint leaves.
- Let it steep for 10 minutes, then strain the herbs.
- Allow the tea to cool before serving.

Dosing Guidelines:

- Small dogs: 1 teaspoon, twice a day.
- Medium dogs: 1 tablespoon, twice a day.
- Large dogs: 2 tablespoons, twice a day.

Tips for Storage:

Refrigerate for up to 3 days. Discard if it develops a sour smell.

Ashwagandha e Honey Anxiety-Relief Tonic

Ashwagandha is an adaptogen that helps reduce stress, and honey adds a touch of sweetness while promoting relaxation.

Ingredients:

- 1/2 teaspoon ashwagandha powder
- 1 teaspoon raw honey
- 1/2 cup water

Instructions:

- Warm the water slightly (do not boil).
- Stir in the ashwagandha powder and honey until dissolved.
- Let it cool before offering it to your dog.

Dosing Guidelines:

- Small dogs: 1 teaspoon, once a day.
- Medium dogs: 1 tablespoon, once a day.
- Large dogs: 2 tablespoons, once a day.

Tips for Storage:

Store in the fridge for up to 2 days. Shake well before use.

Valerian Root e Chamomile Tonic

Valerian root and chamomile make a powerful combination to calm an anxious dog. This tonic can be added to food or served directly.

Ingredients:

- 1/2 teaspoon valerian root powder
- 1 teaspoon dried chamomile flowers
- 1/2 cup water

Instructions:

- Boil water and add valerian root and chamomile.
- Let it simmer for 10 minutes, then strain.
- Allow the liquid to cool before serving.

Dosing Guidelines:

- Small dogs: 1 teaspoon, once a day.
- Medium dogs: 1 tablespoon, once a day.
- Large dogs: 2 tablespoons, once a day.

Tips for Storage:

- Keep refrigerated for up to 3 days. Discard if it changes color or odor.

Skullcap e Lavender Anti-Anxiety Tonic

Skullcap and lavender work together to calm nerves and reduce anxiety in dogs. This tonic is perfect for dogs prone to stress or anxiety.

Ingredients:
- 1/2 teaspoon skullcap powder
- 1 teaspoon dried lavender flowers
- 1/2 cup water

Instructions:
- Boil water and remove from heat.
- Add skullcap powder and lavender flowers to the water.
- Let it steep for 10 minutes, then strain.
- Cool the tonic completely before serving.

Dosing Guidelines:
- Small dogs: 1 teaspoon, once a day.
- Medium dogs: 1 tablespoon, once a day.
- Large dogs: 2 tablespoons, once a day.

Tips for Storage:
Store in a sealed container in the fridge for up to 3 days. Shake before use.
These teas and tonics provide a natural and gentle way to help your dog relax and reduce anxiety. Always consult with your veterinarian before introducing new herbs into your dog's diet.

JOINT AND MOBILITY SUPPORT RECIPES

As dogs age, maintaining joint health becomes increasingly important to ensure mobility and comfort. Inflammation and stiffness in the joints can lead to pain, making it harder for your dog to move around freely. Homemade anti-inflammatory pastes, packed with herbs like turmeric and ginger, provide natural relief for joint pain and arthritis. These easy-to-make recipes promote joint health and reduce inflammation, offering your dog a more active, pain-free life. Always consult your vet before introducing new supplements.

Homemade Anti-Inflammatory Paste

Anti-inflammatory pastes made with herbs like turmeric, ginger, and boswellia can provide natural relief for dogs suffering from joint pain, arthritis, or other inflammatory conditions. These simple homemade recipes help reduce inflammation, promote joint health, and improve overall wellness. The combination of ingredients like black pepper and oils enhances the absorption of turmeric's active compound, curcumin, making these pastes even more effective. Always consult your veterinarian before introducing new supplements into your dog's diet to ensure safety and proper dosage.

Ginger e Turmeric Anti-Inflammatory Paste

This paste combines the powerful anti-inflammatory properties of both ginger and turmeric to help ease joint pain and reduce inflammation.

Ingredients:

- 1/4 cup turmeric powder
- 1 tablespoon grated fresh ginger
- 1/2 cup water
- 1 tablespoon coconut oil
- 1/2 teaspoon ground black pepper

Instructions:

- Mix turmeric powder, ginger, and water in a saucepan.
- Simmer on low heat until it forms a thick paste (about 10 minutes).
- Remove from heat and stir in coconut oil and black pepper.
- Let it cool before serving.

Dosing Guidelines:

- Small dogs: 1/4 teaspoon, once a day.
- Medium dogs: 1/2 teaspoon, once a day.
- Large dogs: 1 teaspoon, once a day.

Tips for Storage:

Store in the fridge for up to 2 weeks in a sealed container.

Green Lipped Mussel e Turmeric Paste

Green-lipped mussel is a natural anti-inflammatory that, when combined with turmeric, helps reduce joint pain and stiffness in dogs.

Ingredients:

- 1/4 cup turmeric powder
- 1 tablespoon green-lipped mussel powder
- 1/2 cup water
- 1 tablespoon olive oil
- 1/2 teaspoon ground black pepper

Instructions:

- Mix turmeric powder, green-lipped mussel powder, and water in a saucepan.
- Simmer on low heat, stirring occasionally, until a thick paste forms.
- Remove from heat and stir in olive oil and black pepper.
- Allow it to cool before serving.

Dosing Guidelines:

- Small dogs: 1/4 teaspoon, once a day.
- Medium dogs: 1/2 teaspoon, once a day.
- Large dogs: 1 teaspoon, once a day.

Tips for Storage:

Keep in the fridge for up to 2 weeks in an airtight container.

Turmeric Golden Paste

This classic anti-inflammatory paste combines turmeric with black pepper and coconut oil to enhance absorption and reduce inflammation in dogs.

Ingredients:

- 1/4 cup turmeric powder
- 1/2 cup water
- 1/4 cup coconut oil
- 1/2 teaspoon ground black pepper

Instructions:

- Mix turmeric powder and water in a saucepan.
- Simmer on low heat, stirring constantly, until a thick paste forms (about 7-10 minutes).
- Remove from heat and stir in the coconut oil and black pepper.
- Allow the paste to cool before serving.

Dosing Guidelines:

- Small dogs: 1/4 teaspoon, once a day.
- Medium dogs: 1/2 teaspoon, once a day.
- Large dogs: 1 teaspoon, once a day.

Tips for Storage:

Store in an airtight container in the refrigerator for up to 2 weeks.

Coconut Oil e Cinnamon Anti-Inflammatory Paste

This simple paste uses the anti-inflammatory benefits of coconut oil and cinnamon to help dogs with joint pain or digestive inflammation.

Ingredients:

- 1/4 cup coconut oil
- 1/2 teaspoon ground cinnamon
- 1/4 cup water

Instructions:

- Warm the coconut oil and water together in a saucepan on low heat.
- Stir in the ground cinnamon until well combined.
- Let the mixture cool and solidify before serving.

Dosing Guidelines:

- Small dogs: 1/4 teaspoon, once a day.
- Medium dogs: 1/2 teaspoon, once a day.
- Large dogs: 1 teaspoon, once a day.

Tips for Storage:

Store in a sealed container in the fridge for up to 2 weeks.

Boswellia e Turmeric Joint Relief Paste

Boswellia is a natural anti-inflammatory herb that supports joint health, and combined with turmeric, this paste helps alleviate pain and stiffness.

Ingredients:

- 1/4 cup turmeric powder
- 1 tablespoon boswellia powder
- 1/2 cup water
- 1 tablespoon coconut oil
- 1/2 teaspoon ground black pepper

Instructions:

- Combine turmeric, boswellia, and water in a saucepan.
- Simmer on low heat, stirring occasionally, until a thick paste forms.
- Remove from heat and stir in the coconut oil and black pepper.
- Let the paste cool before serving.

Dosing Guidelines:

- Small dogs: 1/4 teaspoon, once a day.
- Medium dogs: 1/2 teaspoon, once a day.
- Large dogs: 1 teaspoon, once a day.

Tips for Storage:

Store in the fridge for up to 2 weeks in a sealed container.

These homemade anti-inflammatory pastes are great for promoting joint health and reducing inflammation. Always consult your vet before adding new herbs or supplements to your dog's diet.

Herbal Sprays and Rubs for Sore Muscles and Joints

Herbal sprays and rubs can provide natural relief for dogs dealing with muscle soreness or joint pain. Ingredients like arnica, lavender, peppermint, and turmeric are known for their anti-inflammatory and pain-relieving properties. These easy-to-make remedies can be massaged into your dog's skin to promote comfort and healing. As always, consult your veterinarian before introducing any new treatments to ensure they are safe and appropriate for your dog's condition.

Arnica e Lavender Soothing Spray

This gentle herbal spray combines arnica and lavender, known for their anti-inflammatory and calming properties, to relieve muscle and joint pain in dogs.

Ingredients:

- 1 tablespoon arnica tincture
- 1 teaspoon lavender essential oil
- 1 cup distilled water

Instructions:

- In a spray bottle, combine arnica tincture, lavender essential oil, and distilled water.
- Shake well before each use.

Dosing Guidelines:

Spray directly onto sore muscles or joints 2-3 times a day. Gently rub into the skin.

Tips for Storage:

Store in a cool, dry place. Shake well before each use. Lasts for up to 1 month.

Peppermint e Chamomile Cooling Spray

Peppermint provides a cooling effect, while chamomile soothes inflammation. This spray is perfect for relieving soreness after exercise or walks.

Ingredients:

- 1 teaspoon peppermint essential oil
- 1 tablespoon chamomile tea (brewed and cooled)
- 1 cup distilled water

Instructions:

- Brew chamomile tea and let it cool.
- Mix the tea, peppermint essential oil, and distilled water in a spray bottle.
- Shake well before use.

Dosing Guidelines:

Spray on affected areas 1-2 times a day. Avoid using it on open wounds.

Tips for Storage:

Store in the refrigerator for up to 2 weeks for added cooling effect. Shake well before use.

Rosemary e Eucalyptus Joint Relief Spray

Rosemary and eucalyptus oils are known for their pain-relieving and anti-inflammatory properties, making this spray ideal for joint discomfort.

Ingredients:

- 1 teaspoon rosemary essential oil
- 1 teaspoon eucalyptus essential oil
- 1 cup distilled water

Instructions:

- In a spray bottle, combine the rosemary and eucalyptus oils with distilled water.
- Shake well to mix.

Dosing Guidelines:

- Spray directly on sore joints 1-2 times a day. Gently massage into the skin.

Tips for Storage:

- Store in a cool, dry place for up to 1 month. Shake well before each use.

Turmeric e Coconut Oil Muscle Rub

This rub uses turmeric's anti-inflammatory properties and coconut oil's soothing effects to relieve muscle stiffness and joint pain.

Ingredients:

- 1 tablespoon turmeric powder
- 1/4 cup coconut oil
- 1 teaspoon ground black pepper

Instructions:

- Melt the coconut oil in a saucepan over low heat.
- Stir in turmeric powder and black pepper.
- Let the mixture cool until it solidifies into a paste.

Dosing Guidelines:

- Rub a small amount on sore muscles or joints 1-2 times a day.

Tips for Storage:

Store in a sealed jar in the refrigerator for up to 2 weeks. Let it soften at room temperature before use.

Ginger e Arnica Joint Relief Rub

This rub combines ginger and arnica to help reduce inflammation and pain in sore joints and muscles.

Ingredients:

- 1 tablespoon arnica oil
- 1 teaspoon grated fresh ginger
- 1/4 cup olive oil

Instructions:

- Heat the olive oil over low heat and add grated ginger.
- Let the mixture simmer for 10 minutes, then remove from heat.
- Strain the oil and stir in arnica oil.
- Let it cool before use.

Dosing Guidelines:

- Apply to the affected area and gently massage 1-2 times a day.

Tips for Storage:

Store in a sealed jar in a cool, dry place for up to 2 weeks.

Cayenne e Olive Oil Pain Relief Rub

Cayenne pepper is known for its pain-relieving effects, and when combined with olive oil, it creates a warming rub to soothe aching joints and muscles.

Ingredients:

- 1 teaspoon cayenne pepper powder
- 1/4 cup olive oil
- 1 tablespoon beeswax (optional for a thicker consistency)

Instructions:

- Heat olive oil over low heat and add cayenne pepper powder.
- Simmer for 10 minutes, then strain the oil.
- If using beeswax, melt it into the oil for a thicker consistency.
- Let the mixture cool before applying.

Dosing Guidelines:

- Massage a small amount onto sore areas 1-2 times a day. Avoid use on broken skin.

Tips for Storage:

Store in a sealed container in a cool, dry place for up to 1 month.
These herbal sprays and rubs provide natural relief for your dog's sore muscles and joints. Always consult your vet before using new treatments on your dog, especially if they have any skin sensitivities.

TOPICAL REMEDIES FOR SKIN ISSUES

Dogs can experience skin irritations from allergies, hot spots, or bug bites, and natural topical remedies can help soothe and heal these issues. Herbal healing balms provide deep hydration, promote skin repair, and offer relief for dry, cracked areas like paws and noses. These easy-to-make balms use gentle ingredients like coconut oil, shea butter, and beeswax. Always consult your vet before applying new treatments and test a small area on your dog's skin to ensure no adverse reactions.

Healing Balms

Herbal balms are a natural way to soothe and protect your dog's skin, paws, and nose. Using ingredients like coconut oil, shea butter, beeswax, and essential oils, these balms provide deep hydration, help heal minor wounds, and offer relief for irritated or dry areas. These easy-to-make balms are designed for common issues like cracked paws, dry noses, hot spots, and minor cuts. Always test a small area of your dog's skin first and consult your vet for persistent issues.

Paw Soother Balm

This balm is designed to heal and soothe cracked, dry, or irritated paws. It contains natural ingredients like coconut oil and shea butter to provide deep hydration and protection.

Ingredients:

- 1/4 cup coconut oil
- 1/4 cup shea butter
- 2 tablespoons beeswax
- 1 tablespoon olive oil
- 5 drops lavender essential oil (optional for calming effect)

Instructions:

- In a double boiler, melt the coconut oil, shea butter, and beeswax together.
- Once melted, remove from heat and stir in olive oil and lavender essential oil.
- Pour the mixture into a small container and let it cool and solidify.

Dosing Guidelines:

Apply a small amount to your dog's paws after walks or before bed.

Tips for Storage:

Store in a cool, dry place for up to 6 months.

Hot Spot Healing Balm

This balm helps heal irritated skin, hot spots, and minor wounds. It contains calendula and coconut oil to promote healing and reduce inflammation.

Ingredients:

- 1/4 cup coconut oil
- 1 tablespoon dried calendula flowers
- 1 tablespoon beeswax
- 5 drops tea tree essential oil (optional)

Instructions:

- Gently heat the coconut oil and calendula flowers in a small pot for 15 minutes to infuse the oil.
- Strain the flowers out of the oil.
- In a double boiler, melt the beeswax and then mix it into the calendula-infused coconut oil.
- Add tea tree essential oil if using, and pour into a container to cool.

Dosing Guidelines:

Apply a small amount to affected areas 1-2 times a day.

Tips for Storage:

Store in a cool place for up to 3 months. Avoid sunlight to prevent melting.

Nose Protection Balm

This balm is ideal for dogs with dry or cracked noses. It uses soothing ingredients like shea butter and olive oil to restore moisture and protect the skin.

Ingredients:

- 1/4 cup shea butter
- 2 tablespoons olive oil
- 1 tablespoon beeswax
- 1 teaspoon vitamin E oil

Instructions:

- In a double boiler, melt shea butter and beeswax together.
- Stir in olive oil and vitamin E oil once melted.
- Pour into a small container and let it cool before use.

Dosing Guidelines:

Gently apply a small amount to your dog's nose 1-2 times daily.

Tips for Storage:

Store in a sealed container for up to 6 months.

Wound Healing Balm

This balm supports healing for minor cuts and wounds, using ingredients like comfrey and beeswax to promote skin regeneration and protect the wound area.

Ingredients:

- 1/4 cup coconut oil
- 1 tablespoon dried comfrey leaves
- 2 tablespoons beeswax
- 5 drops tea tree essential oil (optional)

Instructions:

- Heat the coconut oil and comfrey leaves over low heat for 15 minutes to infuse.
- Strain the leaves and return the oil to the heat.
- Melt the beeswax into the infused oil and stir until combined.
- Add tea tree oil and pour into a container to cool.

Dosing Guidelines:

Apply a thin layer to wounds 1-2 times a day.

Tips for Storage:

Store in a cool, dry place for up to 3 months.

Skin Relief Balm

This balm helps soothe itchy, irritated skin caused by allergies or dryness. It contains calming herbs like chamomile and moisturizing ingredients like shea butter.

Ingredients:

- 1/4 cup shea butter
- 2 tablespoons olive oil
- 1 tablespoon dried chamomile flowers
- 1 tablespoon beeswax

Instructions:

- Heat olive oil and chamomile flowers over low heat for 15 minutes to infuse.
- Strain out the flowers and melt the shea butter and beeswax into the infused oil.
- Stir until well combined and pour into a container to cool.

Dosing Guidelines:

Apply to irritated skin 1-2 times a day.

Tips for Storage:

Store in a cool, dry place for up to 6 months.

These healing balms are natural remedies to help your dog with various skin, nose, and paw issues. Always test a small area of your dog's skin before regular use and consult your vet if irritation persists.

Herbal Shampoos and Sprays for Skin Irritations

Herbal shampoos and sprays provide a natural way to soothe your dog's skin irritations, whether caused by allergies, dry skin, or minor infections. These blends use ingredients like oatmeal, aloe, chamomile, tea tree, and lavender to hydrate, heal, and reduce inflammation. When using these natural remedies, always test a small patch of your dog's skin to ensure they don't have any adverse reactions. Consult your veterinarian if skin issues persist or worsen after treatment.

Oatmeal e Aloe Soothing Shampoo

This gentle shampoo is designed to relieve itching and soothe irritated skin. Oatmeal helps reduce inflammation, while aloe vera hydrates and heals.

Ingredients:

- 1/2 cup ground oatmeal
- 1/4 cup aloe vera gel
- 1 tablespoon olive oil
- 1 cup water

Instructions:

- Mix the ground oatmeal, aloe vera gel, and olive oil in a bowl.
- Gradually add the water, stirring until well blended.
- Pour the mixture into a squeeze bottle for easy use.

Dosing Guidelines:

Use during bath time. Massage into your dog's wet coat and let sit for 5-10 minutes before rinsing thoroughly.

Tips for Storage:

Store in a cool, dry place. Use within 1 week, or refrigerate for up to 2 weeks.

Chamomile e Lavender Healing Shampoo

This calming shampoo combines chamomile and lavender to soothe irritated skin and promote healing, making it ideal for dogs with sensitive or inflamed skin.

Ingredients:

- 1/4 cup liquid castile soap
- 1/4 cup brewed chamomile tea (cooled)
- 1 teaspoon lavender essential oil
- 1 tablespoon coconut oil

Instructions:

- Brew the chamomile tea and allow it to cool.
- Mix the tea with liquid castile soap, lavender oil, and coconut oil.
- Shake or stir well to combine.

Dosing Guidelines:

Use during bath time. Lather onto your dog's coat and let it sit for 5 minutes before rinsing.

Tips for Storage:

Store in a sealed bottle for up to 2 weeks in a cool, dry place.

Tea Tree e Neem Anti-Itch Shampoo

Tea tree and neem oil are powerful anti-inflammatory and antimicrobial agents, making this shampoo great for treating skin irritations, infections, and itchiness.

Ingredients:

- 1/4 cup liquid castile soap
- 1 teaspoon tea tree oil
- 1 teaspoon neem oil
- 1 cup distilled water

Instructions:

- In a bottle, combine the castile soap, tea tree oil, and neem oil.
- Add the distilled water and shake to mix well.

Dosing Guidelines:

Apply during bath time. Massage into the coat and allow it to sit for 5 minutes before rinsing thoroughly.

Tips for Storage:

Store in a cool, dry place for up to 2 weeks. Shake well before use.

Apple Cider Vinegar e Aloe Skin Soothing Spray

Apple cider vinegar helps balance skin pH and reduce inflammation, while aloe vera soothes and hydrates the skin, relieving irritation.

Ingredients:

- 1/2 cup apple cider vinegar
- 1/4 cup aloe vera gel
- 1/2 cup distilled water

Instructions:

- In a spray bottle, combine the apple cider vinegar, aloe vera gel, and water.
- Shake well before use.

Dosing Guidelines:

Spray directly on irritated skin 1-2 times a day. Avoid open wounds or eyes.

Tips for Storage:

Store in the refrigerator for up to 2 weeks. Shake well before each use.

Calendula e Chamomile Healing Spray

Calendula is known for its skin-healing properties, and chamomile reduces inflammation and soothes irritated skin. This spray is ideal for minor skin irritations.

Ingredients:

- 1 tablespoon dried calendula flowers
- 1 tablespoon dried chamomile flowers
- 1 cup distilled water

Instructions:

- Boil the water and add calendula and chamomile flowers.
- Let the mixture steep for 15 minutes, then strain.
- Pour the liquid into a spray bottle and let it cool completely.

Dosing Guidelines:

Spray on irritated areas 2-3 times a day to soothe skin.

Tips for Storage:

Store in the fridge for up to 1 week. Shake well before use.

Lavender & Witch Hazel Anti-Itch Spray

Lavender oil calms the skin and reduces itching, while witch hazel acts as an astringent to help heal irritated skin.

Ingredients:

- 1 teaspoon lavender essential oil
- 1/2 cup witch hazel
- 1/2 cup distilled water

Instructions:

- Mix lavender oil, witch hazel, and distilled water in a spray bottle.
- Shake well before each use.

Dosing Guidelines:

Spray directly on irritated areas 1-2 times a day. Avoid the eyes and open wounds.

Tips for Storage:

Store in a cool, dry place for up to 1 month. Shake well before use.

These herbal shampoos and sprays are natural remedies to soothe your dog's skin irritations. Always test a small area of your dog's skin before applying a new treatment, and consult your vet if irritation persists.

DETOXIFICATION RECIPES

Detoxification is essential for removing toxins and supporting your dog's liver and kidney health. Regular, gentle detox recipes can help your dog feel its best by promoting organ function and overall well-being. Liver-cleansing smoothies, made with ingredients like dandelion, beets, turmeric, and parsley, are rich in antioxidants and vitamins to support detoxification. These easy-to-make recipes provide natural detoxification while promoting liver and kidney health. Always consult your veterinarian before introducing new foods or supplements into your dog's diet.

Liver Cleansing Smoothies

Liver-cleansing smoothies made with nutrient-rich ingredients like dandelion, beets, turmeric, and parsley provide a gentle detox and support for your dog's liver. These smoothies are packed with vitamins, antioxidants, and natural detoxifiers that help promote liver health and flush out toxins. Always consult your veterinarian before introducing new foods or supplements into your dog's diet to ensure they're safe and appropriate for their health needs.

Rosemary & Eucalyptus Joint Relief Spray

Rosemary and eucalyptus oils are known for their pain-relieving and anti-inflammatory properties, making this spray ideal for joint discomfort.

Ingredients:

- 1 teaspoon rosemary essential oil
- 1 teaspoon eucalyptus essential oil
- 1 cup distilled water

Instructions:

- In a spray bottle, combine the rosemary and eucalyptus oils with distilled water.
- Shake well to mix.

Dosing Guidelines:

- Spray directly on sore joints 1-2 times a day. Gently massage into the skin.

Tips for Storage:

- Store in a cool, dry place for up to 1 month. Shake well before each use.

Dandelion e Carrot Detox Smoothie

Dandelion is known for its liver-cleansing properties, and when paired with carrots, it provides a vitamin-rich smoothie that supports liver function.

Ingredients:
- 1/2 cup dandelion greens (washed)
- 1/4 cup grated carrots
- 1/4 cup unsweetened coconut water
- 1 tablespoon flaxseed oil

Instructions:
- Combine dandelion greens, carrots, coconut water, and flaxseed oil in a blender.
- Blend until smooth.
- Add more coconut water if needed for consistency.

Dosing Guidelines:
Small dogs: 1 tablespoon, once a day.
Medium dogs: 2 tablespoons, once a day.
Large dogs: 1/4 cup, once a day.

Tips for Storage:
Store in the refrigerator for up to 24 hours. Shake well before serving.

Beet e Spinach Liver Cleanse Smoothie

Beets are packed with antioxidants that promote liver health, and spinach adds additional nutrients to help detoxify the liver.

Ingredients:
- 1/4 cup cooked and cooled beets (diced)
- 1/4 cup fresh spinach
- 1/4 cup unsweetened coconut water
- 1 teaspoon olive oil

Instructions:
- Place beets, spinach, coconut water, and olive oil in a blender.
- Blend until smooth.
- Adjust consistency by adding more coconut water if needed.

Dosing Guidelines:
- Small dogs: 1 tablespoon, once a day.
- Medium dogs: 2 tablespoons, once a day.
- Large dogs: 1/4 cup, once a day.

Tips for Storage:
Store in a sealed container in the refrigerator for up to 24 hours.

Turmeric e Apple Liver Support Smoothie

Turmeric has potent anti-inflammatory and liver-detoxifying effects, while apple provides fiber and essential vitamins for overall liver health.

Ingredients:

- 1/4 teaspoon ground turmeric
- 1/4 cup unsweetened applesauce
- 1/4 cup unsweetened coconut water
- 1 teaspoon flaxseed oil

Instructions:

- Combine turmeric, applesauce, coconut water, and flaxseed oil in a blender.
- Blend until smooth.
- Add water if needed to reach the desired consistency.

Dosing Guidelines:

- Small dogs: 1 tablespoon, once a day.
- Medium dogs: 2 tablespoons, once a day.
- Large dogs: 1/4 cup, once a day.

Tips for Storage:

Store in the fridge for up to 24 hours. Shake or stir well before serving.

Parsley e Cucumber Liver Detox Smoothie

Parsley acts as a natural diuretic, helping to flush toxins from the liver, while cucumber hydrates and provides essential vitamins.

Ingredients:

- 1/4 cup fresh parsley (chopped)
- 1/4 cup cucumber (peeled and diced)
- 1/4 cup water
- 1 teaspoon olive oil

Instructions:

- Blend parsley, cucumber, water, and olive oil until smooth.
- Add more water if needed to adjust the consistency.

Dosing Guidelines:

- Small dogs: 1 tablespoon, once a day.
- Medium dogs: 2 tablespoons, once a day.
- Large dogs: 1/4 cup, once a day.

Tips for Storage:

Store in the refrigerator for up to 24 hours. Shake well before use.

Broccoli e Blueberry Liver Cleansing Smoothie

Broccoli is rich in fiber and antioxidants, while blueberries provide additional liver-supporting nutrients to help detoxify and cleanse.

Ingredients:
- 1/4 cup steamed and cooled broccoli
- 1/4 cup fresh blueberries
- 1/4 cup unsweetened coconut water
- 1 tablespoon flaxseed oil

Instructions:
- Blend broccoli, blueberries, coconut water, and flaxseed oil until smooth.
- Adjust consistency with additional coconut water if needed.

Dosing Guidelines:
- Small dogs: 1 tablespoon, once a day.
- Medium dogs: 2 tablespoons, once a day.
- Large dogs: 1/4 cup, once a day.

Tips for Storage:
Keep in the refrigerator for up to 24 hours. Stir well before serving.
These liver-cleansing smoothies provide natural and gentle detox support for dogs, promoting overall liver health. Always consult your vet before adding new ingredients to your dog's diet.

Gentle Kidney Detox

Kidney health is essential for flushing out toxins and maintaining overall well-being. These gentle kidney detox recipes use natural ingredients like dandelion, parsley, nettle, and celery, which act as diuretics and detoxifiers, supporting healthy kidney function. These homemade remedies provide hydration and help cleanse your dog's kidneys while also being easy to prepare. As always, consult your veterinarian before adding new supplements or herbs to ensure safety and efficacy for your dog's specific needs.

Dandelion e Parsley Kidney Cleanse

Dandelion and parsley are natural diuretics that help promote healthy kidney function by flushing out toxins and supporting detoxification.

Ingredients:
- 1/4 cup fresh dandelion greens (chopped)
- 1/4 cup fresh parsley (chopped)
- 1 cup water

Instructions:
- Boil the water, then remove from heat.
- Add the dandelion greens and parsley to the hot water.
- Let it steep for 10 minutes, then strain.
- Allow it to cool before serving.

Dosing Guidelines:
- Small dogs: 1 teaspoon, once a day.
- Medium dogs: 1 tablespoon, once a day.
- Large dogs: 2 tablespoons, once a day.

Tips for Storage:
Store in the fridge for up to 2 days. Shake well before each use.

Nettle e Cucumber Hydration Detox

Nettle is known for its kidney-supporting properties, while cucumber provides hydration and mild detoxification to help cleanse the kidneys gently.

Ingredients:

- 1 teaspoon dried nettle leaves
- 1/4 cup cucumber (peeled and diced)
- 1 cup water

Instructions:

- Boil water and remove from heat.
- Add nettle leaves and let it steep for 10 minutes, then strain.
- Blend the nettle tea with cucumber until smooth.
- Cool before serving.

Dosing Guidelines:

- Small dogs: 1 teaspoon, once a day.
- Medium dogs: 1 tablespoon, once a day.
- Large dogs: 2 tablespoons, once a day.

Tips for Storage:

Store in the refrigerator for up to 2 days.

Marshmallow Root e Cranberry Kidney Support

Marshmallow root helps soothe and protect the urinary tract, while cranberry supports kidney health by preventing bacterial growth.

Ingredients:

- 1/4 teaspoon marshmallow root powder
- 1 tablespoon unsweetened cranberry juice
- 1 cup water

Instructions:

- Heat water and add marshmallow root powder, stirring until dissolved.
- Allow it to cool, then stir in the cranberry juice.
- Serve cool.

Dosing Guidelines:

- Small dogs: 1 teaspoon, once a day.
- Medium dogs: 1 tablespoon, once a day.
- Large dogs: 2 tablespoons, once a day.

Tips for Storage:

Store in the fridge for up to 2 days. Shake well before use.

Celery e Apple Kidney Detox Drink

Celery acts as a natural diuretic, helping flush toxins from the kidneys, while apple provides antioxidants to support overall kidney health.

Ingredients:
- 1/4 cup chopped celery
- 1/4 cup unsweetened applesauce
- 1 cup water

Instructions:
- Blend celery and applesauce with water until smooth.
- Strain to remove any chunks if needed.
- Let it cool before serving.

Dosing Guidelines:
- Small dogs: 1 teaspoon, once a day.
- Medium dogs: 1 tablespoon, once a day.
- Large dogs: 2 tablespoons, once a day.

Tips for Storage:
Store in the fridge for up to 2 days. Stir before serving.

Burdock Root e Dandelion Detox Tonic

Overview: Burdock root and dandelion support the kidneys by flushing out toxins and enhancing overall kidney function, making this a gentle detox tonic.

Ingredients:
- 1/4 teaspoon dried burdock root
- 1/4 cup fresh dandelion greens
- 1 cup water

Instructions:
- Boil water and add burdock root and dandelion greens.
- Simmer for 10 minutes, then strain.
- Let it cool completely before offering it to your dog.

Dosing Guidelines:
- Small dogs: 1 teaspoon, once a day.
- Medium dogs: 1 tablespoon, once a day.
- Large dogs: 2 tablespoons, once a day.

Tips for Storage:
Keep in the refrigerator for up to 2 days.
These gentle kidney detox recipes provide natural ways to support your dog's kidney health. Always consult your vet before introducing new herbs or supplements into your dog's diet.

ALTERNATIVE NATURAL REMEDIES BEYOND HERBS

While herbs are a cornerstone of natural healing for dogs, they're not the only option. Other remedies, such as aromatherapy, flower essences, and superfoods, can also play a significant role in your dog's health journey. Let's explore how you can incorporate alternative natural remedies into your dog's care.

Aromatherapy and Essential Oils for Dogs

Aromatherapy can be a powerful tool for calming your dog, promoting healing, and even repelling pests. However, it's crucial to understand that not all essential oils are safe for dogs, and even safe oils must be used carefully. Below are five essential oils that are safe for use in aromatherapy for dogs, along with guidelines for how to use them safely and important precautions.

LAVENDER ESSENTIAL OIL

Lavender is one of the most versatile and safest essential oils for dogs. It has calming properties that can help reduce anxiety, stress, and restlessness, especially during thunderstorms or vet visits.

How to Use: Dilute lavender oil in a 1% solution (1 drop of essential oil to 100 drops of carrier oil like coconut or olive oil). You can apply it to your dog's bedding or use it in a diffuser for a calming environment.

Precautions: Ensure proper ventilation when diffusing lavender oil, and avoid applying it directly to your dog's skin. Always observe your dog for any signs of irritation or discomfort when first using lavender.

CHAMOMILE ESSENTIAL OIL

Chamomile oil is gentle and calming, perfect for dogs that are anxious or suffer from digestive issues. Its anti-inflammatory properties can also soothe skin irritations.

How to Use: Dilute in a 1% solution and apply to a bandana or bedding, or add a few drops to a diffuser. You can also mix it with a carrier oil and apply it to areas of minor skin irritation.

Precautions: Avoid using chamomile oil near your dog's face, especially around their eyes, nose, and mouth. If ingested, it may cause mild stomach upset, so keep the oil out of your dog's reach.

FRANKINCENSE ESSENTIAL OIL

Frankincense has healing properties that can support immune function, reduce inflammation, and promote emotional well-being. It's a great choice for older dogs or those recovering from illness.

How to Use: Dilute in a carrier oil and massage it gently onto your dog's chest or back. You can also diffuse it to create a calming environment, especially during stressful events.

Precautions: Avoid direct contact with sensitive areas like the eyes or open wounds. Always use a diluted form of frankincense and monitor your dog's response.

CEDARWOOD ESSENTIAL OIL

Cedarwood oil is known for its insect-repellent properties and can help prevent fleas and ticks. It also has a grounding and calming effect, making it useful for anxious dogs.

How to Use: Dilute in a 1% solution and apply to your dog's collar or bedding. Alternatively, you can diffuse it in your home to create an insect-repellent environment.

Precautions: Cedarwood oil should not be used on puppies or pregnant dogs. Avoid using it directly on your dog's skin unless diluted, and never apply it near your dog's eyes or mucous membranes.

GINGER ESSENTIAL OIL

Ginger oil is beneficial for dogs suffering from nausea or digestive issues. Its warming properties can also help relieve joint pain in older dogs.

How to Use: Dilute ginger oil and massage it gently into areas where your dog experiences discomfort, or diffuse it in small amounts if your dog tends to get car sick.

Precautions: Always dilute ginger oil before use, and avoid using it on dogs with sensitive skin. Never let your dog ingest the oil, as it can be toxic in large quantities.

GENERAL SAFETY TIPS

Dilution: Always dilute essential oils to a 1% solution before use. Essential oils are potent, and even safe oils can cause harm if used incorrectly.

Application: Do not apply essential oils directly to your dog's skin, and avoid letting them lick the oils. Diffusion or topical application with a carrier oil is the safest approach.

Consult a Vet: Always consult with your veterinarian before using any essential oils on your dog, especially if they have underlying health conditions.

By following these guidelines, you can safely incorporate essential oils into your dog's wellness routine while minimizing any risks.

Flower Essences and Their Role in Emotional Healing

Flower essences are a subtle form of natural remedy that works on your dog's emotional and behavioral well-being. Unlike essential oils, flower essences are completely safe to use internally and externally, making them ideal for sensitive dogs. Each essence targets specific emotional imbalances and can help with a variety of behavioral issues.

RESCUE REMEDY

Rescue Remedy is one of the most well-known flower essence blends. It is often used to help dogs cope with stress, anxiety, or traumatic experiences, such as visits to the vet, thunderstorms, or separation anxiety.

How it works: Rescue Remedy is a blend of five different flower essences designed to calm and reassure dogs during times of stress. It can be added to your dog's water bowl, dropped onto their tongue, or rubbed onto their ears or paws.

Precautions: While generally safe, always follow the recommended dosage. Watch for signs of allergic reactions, such as skin irritation or upset stomach, though these are rare.

MIMULUS

Mimulus flower essence is particularly useful for dogs that display fear of specific things, such as loud noises, strangers, or new environments. It helps dogs become more confident and less anxious in the face of their fears.

How it works: Mimulus works by gently reducing fear and helping your dog feel more secure in situations that typically cause them stress. It can be administered by adding a few drops to your dog's water or food.

Precautions: As with all flower essences, avoid overuse. Introduce it gradually and monitor your dog's behavior to ensure it's providing the desired calming effect.

WALNUT

Walnut flower essence is known for helping dogs adjust to change, such as moving to a new home, the arrival of a new pet, or other major life transitions. It supports emotional resilience and adaptability.

How it works: Walnut essence helps dogs emotionally transition through new or challenging situations by providing stability and comfort. It can be applied directly to their fur or added to their food or water.

Precautions: Start with small doses and gradually increase if necessary. If your dog shows no improvement after prolonged use, consider consulting a holistic veterinarian.

STAR OF BETHLEHEM

This flower essence is ideal for dogs that have experienced trauma, whether physical or emotional. It is often used to comfort rescue dogs or those who have been in accidents or abuse situations.

How it works: Star of Bethlehem helps alleviate shock, grief, and trauma by soothing emotional pain and promoting recovery. It can be given directly by mouth, applied to the skin, or added to your dog's drinking water. It's important to note that while the Star of Bethlehem plant is toxic and dangerous if ingested, the Star of Bethlehem Bach flower essence is completely safe for dogs. The preparation method eliminates any toxic compounds, making it safe to use for emotional healing.

Precautions: While highly beneficial, it's important to observe your dog for any changes in behavior, as emotional healing can take time. Avoid using it as a replacement for professional veterinary care if your dog has ongoing behavioral issues.

ASPEN

Aspen flower essence is used for dogs with generalized anxiety or those who seem uneasy for no obvious reason. It helps bring about a sense of calm and reduces underlying nervousness.

How it works: Aspen works by calming dogs that are anxious, especially those that appear to have constant worry or fear of the unknown. A few drops can be added to their food or water, or applied directly to their skin.

Precautions: Always use flower essences in moderation, and observe your dog for any behavioral changes. If anxiety persists, consult your veterinarian for further advice.

GENERAL GUIDELINES FOR USING FLOWER ESSENCES

Dosage: Flower essences are safe and gentle, but it's still important to follow recommended guidelines. Generally, 2-4 drops can be added to your dog's water or directly to their skin.

Application: You can administer flower essences by adding them to food or water, applying them to your dog's fur, or placing drops on their paws or ears.

Consult a Vet: Although flower essences are safe, always consult your veterinarian, especially if your dog has underlying health issues or is on medication.

Flower essences offer a gentle and natural way to support your dog's emotional well-being, helping them find balance and comfort through life's challenges.

Superfoods and Natural Supplements for Enhanced Health

In addition to herbs, certain superfoods and natural supplements can offer your dog an extra boost of nutrients, antioxidants, and immune support. Here are six superfoods and supplements that can contribute to your dog's overall well-being.

TURMERIC

Turmeric is a powerful anti-inflammatory that can help reduce joint pain, making it especially beneficial for dogs with arthritis or other inflammatory conditions. It also supports liver function and overall health.

How to Use: Turmeric is safe in small doses and can be mixed into your dog's food. Start with about 1/8 teaspoon per 10 pounds of your dog's weight, and increase gradually.

Precautions: Ensure your dog is well-hydrated, as turmeric can cause constipation if not taken with enough water. Also, consult your vet before use if your dog has any underlying health conditions.

COCONUT OIL

Rich in healthy fats, coconut oil can support skin health, improve digestion, and boost energy levels. It's also great for promoting a shiny coat and preventing dry, itchy skin.

How to Use: Start with a small amount, such as a quarter teaspoon for small dogs, and gradually increase if tolerated. You can mix it into your dog's food or apply it topically for skin health.

Precautions: Too much coconut oil can lead to diarrhea or weight gain, so always introduce it gradually and in moderation.

SPIRULINA

Spirulina is a nutrient-dense superfood packed with protein, vitamins, and minerals. It's particularly effective in strengthening the immune system, detoxifying the body, and promoting healthy aging in older dogs.

How to Use: Spirulina is available in powder form and can be sprinkled onto your dog's food. About 1/4 teaspoon for small dogs and 1 teaspoon for larger dogs is usually recommended.

Precautions: Make sure to source high-quality spirulina, free from contaminants. Consult your vet before use, particularly if your dog has liver or kidney issues.

BLUEBERRIES

Blueberries are a fantastic source of antioxidants, which help protect your dog's cells from damage and support a healthy immune system. They're also rich in fiber and vitamin C.

How to Use: You can offer blueberries as a snack or mix them into your dog's meals. About 5-10 blueberries a day for small dogs and 10-20 for larger dogs is generally safe.

Precautions: Although rare, some dogs may be allergic to blueberries. Introduce them slowly and observe for any signs of allergic reactions such as itching or digestive upset.

PUMPKIN

Pumpkin is a fiber-rich superfood that helps regulate digestion and can soothe both diarrhea and constipation. It's also packed with beta-carotene, which supports eye health and boosts the immune system.

How to Use: Canned, unsweetened pumpkin is the easiest way to serve it to your dog. Start with 1 tablespoon per 10 pounds of body weight, mixed into their food.

Precautions: Ensure you are using plain pumpkin without added sugar or spices. Overuse can cause loose stools, so stick to small amounts.

FISH OIL

Fish oil is rich in omega-3 fatty acids, which help reduce inflammation, support heart health, improve cognitive function, and promote a healthy coat. It's especially useful for dogs with arthritis or skin conditions.

How to Use: You can find fish oil in capsule or liquid form. Add it to your dog's food according to their weight—usually about 20 mg per pound of body weight.

Precautions: Make sure the fish oil you use is specifically formulated for dogs, and avoid giving too much, as it can cause digestive upset or imbalance in omega-6 fatty acids.

GENERAL GUIDELINES FOR USING SUPERFOODS AND SUPPLEMENTS

Dosage: Always follow the recommended dosage and introduce new foods gradually to ensure your dog tolerates them well.

Quality: Choose high-quality, organic options whenever possible to avoid contaminants or additives that could harm your dog.

Consult a Vet: Before introducing any new supplement or superfood, consult with your veterinarian, especially if your dog has pre-existing health conditions or is on medication.

By incorporating these superfoods and natural supplements into your dog's diet, you can support their health naturally while boosting their immune system, promoting joint health, and improving digestion.

THE BOTTOM LINE

In this chapter, you explored simple, natural remedies you can easily make at home to support your dog's health. From everyday wellness recipes to digestive health support, calming solutions, joint care, and skin treatments, you now have practical tools to help your dog feel their best. Each recipe was designed to be easy to follow, even if you're new to herbal remedies, with clear steps and safe dosages to keep things stress-free.

By trying out these recipes, you can create personalized care for your dog, naturally supporting their health. Remember, every dog is unique, so feel free to adjust the recipes to suit their specific needs, but always follow the guidelines carefully.

Special Considerations and Advanced Practices

CHAPTER 6

Advanced herbal practices for dogs involve combining specific herbs to address multiple health concerns, but this should be done under the supervision of a qualified herbalist or veterinarian to avoid adverse interactions." – Dr. Richard Pitcairn

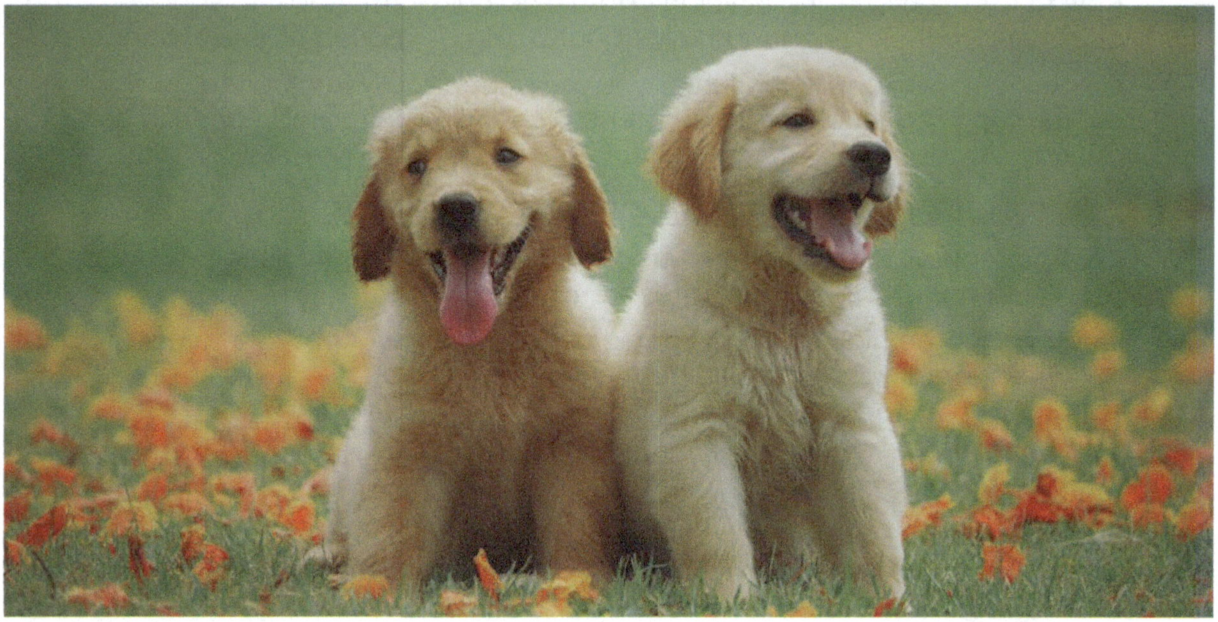

When it comes to caring for your dog's health, you've likely explored basic herbal remedies, such as using chamomile to soothe anxiety or peppermint for digestion. But what happens when your dog has special needs—such as pregnancy, chronic health conditions, or specific recovery goals? This is where you step into more advanced territory, learning how to tailor herbal care to fit your dog's unique circumstances. By mastering these practices, you can give your dog the best possible support and even integrate these remedies with nutritional strategies for holistic well-being.

This chapter is for the dog owner who wants to deepen their understanding of herbal remedies, especially for special populations of dogs, and to enhance the healing potential through thoughtful nutrition. Whether your dog is pregnant, a growing puppy, or managing a chronic condition, this chapter will guide you through the nuances of herbal care. Let's dive into the world of advanced herbal practices for dogs and discover how you can take their health journey to the next level.

HERBAL REMEDIES FOR SPECIAL DOG POPULATIONS

When using herbal remedies, one size doesn't fit all. Dogs in different stages of life or with unique health challenges require a tailored approach. The goal is to support their healing and well-being while being mindful of their specific needs.

Pregnant and Nursing Dogs

Pregnancy is a delicate time, not just for human moms but for dogs as well. A dog's body is going through significant changes, and while herbal remedies can be helpful, they need to be used with extra caution. Some herbs that may be perfectly safe for a regular adult dog might pose risks during pregnancy.

For example, herbs like raspberry leaf are known for their ability to tone the uterine muscles and may be beneficial in the later stages of pregnancy, supporting smoother labor. According to herbal experts, raspberry leaf can be a gentle but effective aid in preparing the body for birth, helping the uterus to contract more efficiently. However, you must be cautious with dosage and avoid herbs that could stimulate premature contractions or miscarriage, such as pennyroyal or parsley.

If your dog is nursing, you can consider herbs that not only help the mother recover but also promote lactation. Fenugreek is commonly used to boost milk production. However, while fenugreek is safe in moderate amounts, too much of it can cause digestive upset in both mother and pups. The key is always moderation and understanding how your dog's body reacts.

Anecdote: One breeder shared that adding a small amount of fenugreek to her dog's food during nursing helped significantly increase the milk supply, ensuring that all the puppies thrived. However, she was careful to monitor her dog for any signs of digestive issues, as fenugreek can cause loose stools in some dogs.

Puppies and Young Dogs

Puppies are growing rapidly, and their systems are still developing, so it's essential to be mindful of how you introduce herbs to their diet. Young dogs typically have more sensitive digestive systems than adult dogs, so you'll want to focus on gentle, supportive herbs.

For instance, chamomile can be a great choice for puppies who are prone to nervousness or digestive upset. Chamomile is known for its calming effects and ability to ease an upset stomach. However, you should administer it in small, diluted doses to avoid overwhelming their system. Puppies don't need much intervention, but herbs like echinacea can help boost their immune system during stressful times like vaccinations or weaning.

A crucial consideration is the potential for allergic reactions. Just like humans, dogs can be allergic to certain herbs, and puppies might be more sensitive. Always introduce one herb at a time and monitor how your puppy responds. If there's any sign of itching, swelling, or digestive upset, discontinue use immediately.

Expert Quote: Dr. Karen Becker, an integrative veterinarian, advises that "herbs can be extremely beneficial for puppies, but it's vital to consult with a holistic vet to ensure the herbs you're using are appropriate for their age and breed."

Dogs with Pre-existing Medical Conditions (Heart, Kidney, etc.)

For dogs with pre-existing medical conditions, herbal remedies can be both helpful and potentially harmful if not used correctly. The goal is to support their condition without interfering with any current treatments or medications they may be on.

Hawthorn is an excellent herbal remedy for dogs with heart conditions. It strengthens the heart and improves circulation without overstimulating the body. However, if your dog is already on heart medication, you'll want to consult a vet to ensure that hawthorn won't interfere with their medication.

Dogs with kidney issues require extra care when using herbs. Dandelion root can help support the kidneys by acting as a gentle diuretic, promoting the elimination of toxins. However, it's crucial to avoid overuse, as excessive diuretics can put too much strain on already weakened kidneys. Milk thistle is another herb that is often used to support liver function, which can also benefit dogs with kidney problems since the liver and kidneys work closely together to detoxify the body.

Research supports the use of milk thistle in managing liver and kidney health. A study published in the "Journal of Veterinary Internal Medicine" showed that milk thistle could help reduce oxidative stress in dogs with liver conditions, which also has a knock-on effect on kidney health.

COMBINING HERBAL REMEDIES WITH NUTRITION FOR DOGS

Herbs are powerful on their own, but when combined with the right nutrition, their healing potential is significantly enhanced. The synergy between a dog's diet and herbal remedies can improve recovery times, boost immunity, and promote overall health.

How Diet Influences Healing and Recovery for Dogs

The old saying "you are what you eat" rings true for your dog too. Nutrition is the foundation of good health, and when your dog is ill or recovering, their diet plays a crucial role in supporting their body's natural healing processes. When you combine this with herbal remedies, you can create a powerful approach to recovery.

A dog recovering from surgery or illness needs a diet rich in antioxidants, vitamins, and minerals to repair tissues, boost the immune system, and prevent inflammation. Foods like sweet potatoes, blueberries, and leafy greens are packed with these nutrients. When paired with anti-inflammatory herbs like turmeric, which contains curcumin and is known for its powerful anti-inflammatory properties, your dog's recovery can be accelerated.

For dogs with digestive issues, adding herbs like slippery elm, which coats and soothes the digestive tract, alongside a diet rich in easy-to-digest foods like bone broth, can make a world of difference. The combination helps heal the gut lining and restores balance, reducing discomfort and promoting a quicker recovery.

Integrating Herbal Supplements with Whole Food Diets for Dogs

Herbs can complement whole foods in your dog's diet, making meals more nutritious and therapeutic. You can think of herbs as a nutritional boost that helps your dog's body get the most out of their food.

For instance, adding herbs like nettle or spirulina to your dog's food can provide a dense source of vitamins and minerals. Nettle is rich in iron and calcium, while spirulina offers a high concentration of protein and antioxidants. These herbs work especially well when added to homemade or raw diets, where whole, unprocessed foods are used.

But how do you integrate these herbs into your dog's diet? One easy method is to create an herbal sprinkle that you can add to their meals. Mix powdered herbs like spirulina, nettle, and turmeric with a bit of coconut oil and sprinkle it over your dog's food. This not only enhances the flavor but also delivers a concentrated dose of health benefits. Finally, slowly introduce new herbs into your dog's diet. Start with small amounts and observe how your dog reacts before gradually increasing the dosage.

ADVANCED HERBAL FORMULATIONS FOR DOGS

Once you have a good grasp of using basic herbs, it's time to explore more advanced herbal formulations. This involves creating custom blends tailored to your dog's specific health goals and choosing the right form for administration.

Creating Custom Blends for Specific Health Goals for Dogs

Creating a custom herbal blend allows you to address multiple health issues at once. For example, if your dog has arthritis and digestive issues, you might combine anti-inflammatory herbs like turmeric with digestive-supporting herbs like ginger and marshmallow root. This blend would not only help reduce pain and inflammation in their joints but also soothe their digestive tract.

When formulating blends, it's important to understand the synergy between herbs. Some herbs work better together than alone, while others may counteract each other's effects. For instance, combining herbs that are both cooling (like peppermint) and warming (like ginger) can create a balanced effect that supports both digestion and circulation.

It's also important to think about your dog's individual constitution. Is your dog more prone to being anxious or lethargic? Are they a high-energy dog, or do they need help calming down? Tailoring herbal blends to fit these traits can make a significant difference in their overall well-being.

Tinctures vs. Capsules vs. Powders: Choosing the Right Form for Dogs

Herbal remedies come in many forms, and each has its advantages depending on your dog's needs. Tinctures, capsules, and powders are the most common, and choosing the right one can influence how effective the remedy is for your dog.

Tinctures are alcohol-based extracts of herbs, and they tend to be more potent than other forms. They're absorbed quickly and are great for dogs who need immediate relief, such as during an anxiety episode or digestive upset. However, the alcohol content might not be ideal for all dogs, especially if they're sensitive or have liver issues. In these cases, glycerin-based tinctures are a better option, offering the same benefits without the alcohol.

Capsules are convenient and easy to measure, making them a good choice if you need to administer a specific dose. They're ideal for long-term use, such as for managing chronic conditions like arthritis or supporting kidney health. However, some dogs may have difficulty swallowing capsules, so you'll need to decide if this method works for your pet.

Powders are versatile and can easily be mixed into your dog's food, making them a popular option. They're especially useful for herbs that have a strong flavor, as mixing them with food helps mask the taste. However, because they're less concentrated than tinctures, you may need to use larger quantities to achieve the same effect.

THE BOTTOM LINE

As we wrap up Chapter 6, you've learned how to tailor herbal remedies for different dogs, whether they're puppies, expecting, or dealing with chronic issues. You also discovered how combining herbs with good nutrition can boost your dog's health even more. Plus, we explored some advanced herbal techniques, like making your own blends and choosing the right form of herbs for your furry friend.

Understanding these special considerations and advanced practices gives you the tools to take your dog's wellness to the next level. You're now equipped to create personalized herbal solutions that fit your dog's unique needs.

But there's more to explore! In Chapter 7, we'll dive into DIY Herbal Projects for Dog Owners. You'll learn fun and easy projects to make your own herbal products at home. From calming treats to immune-boosting teas, these projects will empower you to take control of your dog's health in creative ways. Get ready to roll up your sleeves and start making natural remedies that you and your dog can both enjoy.

Stay tuned for practical tips and step-by-step guides that will make herbal crafting simple and enjoyable. Your journey to a healthier, happier dog continues with exciting new possibilities. Let's move forward and discover how you can become a DIY herbal pro for your beloved pet!

DIY Herbal Projects for Dog Owners

CHAPTER 7

"By preparing your own herbal treatments at home, you ensure that your dog is getting fresh, high-quality ingredients tailored specifically to their needs." – Mary L. Wulff

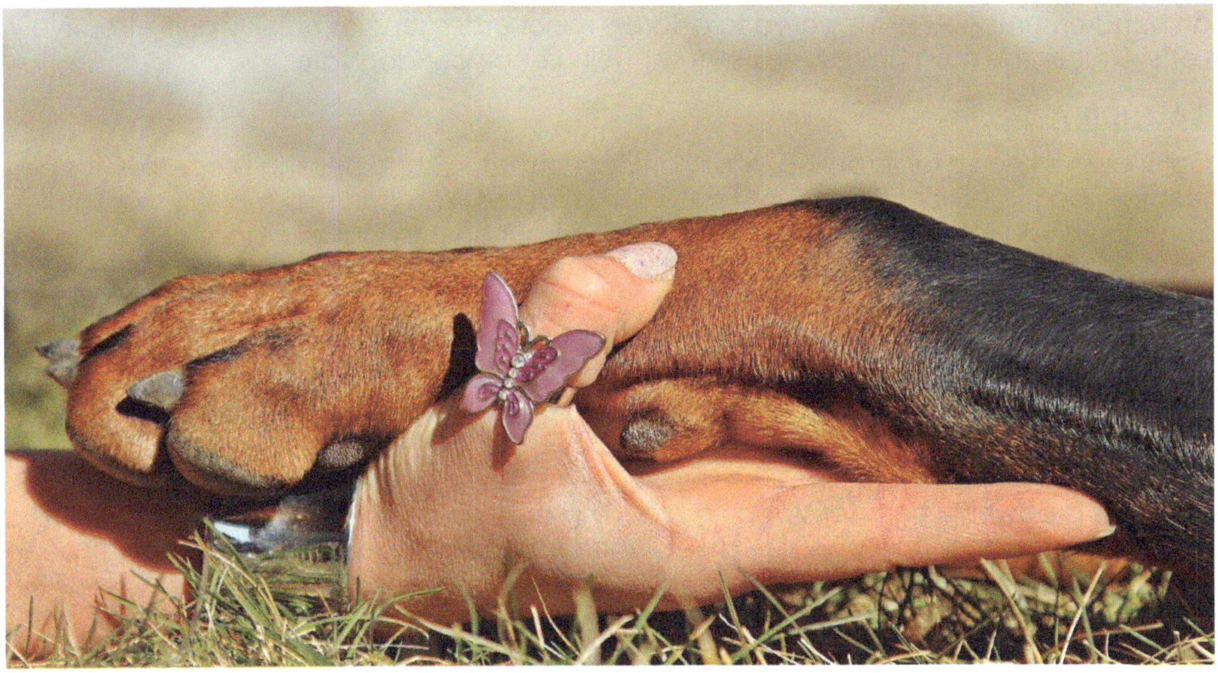

As a dog owner, you know that your furry companion depends on you for everything—from love and companionship to proper care and well-being. When it comes to their health, there's nothing quite as empowering as being able to take matters into your own hands with natural, safe remedies that can help your dog thrive. Have you ever thought about the power of herbs and how they can be part of your dog's health routine? DIY herbal projects not only allow you to address common issues your dog may face but also provide an opportunity to bond and care for them in a more holistic way.

Imagine having a homemade herbal first-aid kit that's always ready for those small emergencies, like a cut on the paw or an insect bite during a walk. Or think about the peace of mind you'll feel knowing you can whip up calming chews for your anxious dog before a vet visit. Herbal remedies are not only effective, but they are also affordable, safe, and customizable to your dog's unique needs. By learning to create herbal solutions at home, you take control of your pet's health, one DIY project at a time. Let's dive into how you can start using herbs to make your dog's life better.

CREATING YOUR OWN HERBAL FIRST-AID KIT

A first-aid kit is an essential tool for every dog owner. Whether your dog spends a lot of time outdoors or is more of an indoor companion, accidents happen. The good news is that many common herbs can be just as effective for dogs as they are for humans. By putting together your own herbal first-aid kit, you'll be well-prepared for any minor emergencies that come your way.

Must-Have Herbs for Common Emergencies

Herbs are a valuable addition to any emergency kit, offering natural remedies for common issues. With their healing, soothing, and immune-boosting properties, these herbs can provide relief from cuts, wounds, digestive problems, and stress. From calendula's antibacterial properties to yarrow's ability to stop bleeding, keeping these essential herbs on hand ensures you're prepared to address minor emergencies quickly and effectively. Let's explore the must-have herbs that will help keep your dog safe.

CALENDULA

Calendula is known for its antibacterial, anti-inflammatory, and healing properties. It's perfect for treating minor cuts, wounds, and skin irritations. You can make a salve or tincture from calendula to apply directly to your dog's skin when they have scrapes or hot spots.

CHAMOMILE

Chamomile is a calming herb with anti-inflammatory properties, making it great for soothing irritated skin and calming upset tummies. It can be used as a wash for minor wounds or added to food as a digestive aid.

YARROW

Yarrow is a powerful herb for stopping bleeding and treating wounds. If your dog gets a small cut or scrape, applying powdered yarrow can help reduce bleeding and speed up the healing process.

LAVENDER

Lavender is known for its calming properties, but it's also an excellent antiseptic. It can be used to clean wounds, soothe burns, and even help reduce anxiety during stressful situations like thunderstorms.

GOLDENSEAL

This herb is a natural antibiotic and can be used for treating infected wounds. A tincture made from goldenseal can be applied to cuts, scrapes, or inflamed areas to prevent infection and promote healing.

SLIPPERY ELM

Slippery elm is excellent for soothing the digestive system. If your dog experiences diarrhea or an upset stomach, mixing slippery elm powder with water to create a paste can help coat the stomach and intestines, reducing irritation and discomfort.

GINGER

Ginger is a great herb for treating nausea, motion sickness, and digestive issues in dogs. You can give your dog small amounts of fresh ginger or add ginger powder to their food to help with vomiting or an upset stomach.

MARSHMALLOW ROOT

Marshmallow root is known for its mucilaginous properties, making it great for soothing irritated tissues. It's useful for soothing sore throats, easing digestive discomfort, and helping with urinary tract infections. You can make a tea or tincture and administer it to your dog for relief.

ECHINACEA

Echinacea is a powerful immune booster that can help your dog fight off infections and illnesses. It can be used to prevent or treat colds, respiratory issues, and even skin infections. A tincture or capsule form is best for giving it to dogs.

PEPPERMINT

Peppermint is another digestive aid and can also help with cooling your dog down. If your dog is overheated or struggling with nausea, a small amount of peppermint tea or tincture can help soothe the stomach and provide cooling relief.

Step-by-Step Guide to Preparing Herbal First-Aid Supplies

Now that you know which herbs to include, it's time to prepare your herbal first-aid kit for your dog. Creating a homemade herbal first-aid kit ensures you are equipped with natural, gentle remedies to handle minor injuries and common health issues like cuts, burns, or digestive discomfort. With just a few basic steps, you can create salves, infusions, and tinctures that offer safe and effective relief. This guide will walk you through gathering the right herbs, crafting versatile treatments, and properly storing them. By preparing these supplies in advance, you'll be ready to provide immediate care whenever your dog needs it.

STEP 1: GATHER YOUR HERBS

The first step in building your herbal first-aid kit is sourcing the right herbs. You can either buy dried herbs from reputable suppliers or, if you prefer, grow your own. Growing your herbs is ideal if you have space and time, as it gives you complete control over the quality and purity of the plants. However, buying dried herbs from trusted sources is just as effective and a good starting point if you're new to herbal remedies.

Ensure that the herbs you purchase or grow are organic and free from pesticides or chemicals, as dogs can be more sensitive to these substances than humans. Popular online stores or health food shops often offer certified organic options. Common herbs like calendula, chamomile, and yarrow are easy to find and great for beginner herbalists.

STEP 2: PREPARE HERBAL INFUSIONS

Infusions are an easy and useful way to extract the healing properties of certain herbs. You can use them as washes for irritated skin or minor wounds or as gentle remedies for digestive issues.

To make an infusion, steep dried or fresh herbs in hot water for 10-15 minutes. Chamomile and lavender, both known for their calming and anti-inflammatory properties, are ideal choices. For instance, you can create a chamomile tea infusion by adding one teaspoon of dried chamomile flowers to a cup of boiling water, letting it steep, and then straining it. Once cooled, this can be applied to minor skin irritations or fed in small amounts to soothe an upset stomach.

Lavender infusion, similarly, can help soothe anxiety or be used as a gentle antiseptic wash for small wounds.

STEP 3: MAKE SALVES AND OINTMENTS

Salves are incredibly versatile and easy to make at home. These thick, balm-like products can be applied to your dog's skin to treat cuts, burns, or dry patches.

Start by gathering beeswax, coconut oil (or olive oil), and your chosen herb (like calendula, known for its healing properties). To make a simple calendula salve, steep a handful of dried calendula flowers in a cup of warm oil for several hours or overnight. Strain the mixture, then combine the infused oil with melted beeswax to create a smooth salve. You can store this in small jars, ready to apply to your dog's minor cuts, scrapes, or dry skin whenever needed.

STEP 4: CREATE TINCTURES

Tinctures are concentrated herbal extracts that can be administered orally or applied topically. They are usually made by soaking herbs in alcohol or glycerin to extract their medicinal properties. For example, a tincture made from goldenseal, a natural antibiotic, can help treat infections in cuts or scrapes. Use a few drops on the affected area to prevent infection. For a more dog-friendly option, glycerin-based tinctures are recommended, as alcohol can be too harsh for pets.

STEP 5: STORE YOUR SUPPLIES

Proper storage is essential to keep your herbal remedies fresh and effective. Store infusions, salves, and tinctures in airtight, labeled containers. Dark glass jars are ideal as they protect the contents from light, which can degrade the herbs over time.

Be sure to label each container with the name of the herb and the date it was made. Most homemade herbal remedies will last for several months if stored in a cool, dark place. If you notice any changes in smell or texture, it's time to make a fresh batch.

STEP 6: USE WHEN NEEDED

Before using any herbal remedy on your dog, it's important to do a patch test. Apply a small amount of the product to a non-sensitive area of your dog's skin to check for any allergic reactions. If no reaction occurs after 24 hours, it's safe to use the remedy as needed.

When applying salves or tinctures, always use clean hands or a cotton ball to avoid introducing bacteria to the wound. For digestive aids like ginger or slippery elm, follow recommended dosages based on your dog's size and weight.

By preparing your herbal first-aid supplies ahead of time, you'll have natural, effective remedies ready to help your dog when they need it most. Whether it's soothing a minor cut or calming a nervous stomach, these herbal treatments offer gentle yet powerful healing solutions for everyday emergencies.

HERBAL HOME REMEDIES FOR COMMON ISSUES

Herbs can provide natural solutions for everyday issues your dog may face, from minor cuts to anxiety. Quick herbal remedies are great for addressing common injuries like scrapes, bites, and irritations, offering gentle yet effective care. Ingredients like calendula, aloe vera, and witch hazel can help soothe wounds and promote healing while cooling sprays made with peppermint and chamomile provide relief on hot days. These simple, natural remedies can help you keep your dog healthy and comfortable.

Quick Fixes for Minor Cuts, Bites, and Scrapes

Dogs are naturally curious, often leading to minor cuts, bites, and scrapes during their adventures. Thankfully, herbal remedies offer effective and gentle solutions for these small injuries. From calendula and aloe vera to soothe cuts to witch hazel for insect bites, using natural ingredients can promote quick healing and prevent infections. In this section, we'll explore easy-to-use herbal fixes, ensuring you're prepared to address your dog's minor wounds with simple yet powerful remedies.

CALENDULA AND ALOE VERA FOR WOUND HEALING

If your dog has a small cut or scrape, a combination of calendula and aloe vera can speed up the healing process. Calendula reduces inflammation and helps the skin repair itself, while aloe vera soothes the area and keeps it moisturized. Apply this mixture as a salve to the affected area twice a day until the wound heals.

WITCH HAZEL FOR BUG BITES

Witch hazel is a natural astringent that helps reduce swelling and itching from insect bites. Simply apply a small amount of witch hazel to the bite using a cotton pad. You can mix it with a few drops of lavender essential oil to increase its soothing effect.

HONEY FOR INFECTION PREVENTION

Raw honey is a natural antibacterial agent that can help prevent infections in minor cuts or scrapes. After cleaning the wound, apply a thin layer of raw honey directly to the affected area. It creates a barrier against bacteria while promoting healing. Reapply as needed until the wound shows signs of healing.

COCONUT OIL FOR SOOTHING IRRITATIONS

Coconut oil has antifungal, antibacterial, and moisturizing properties, making it a great remedy for scrapes and skin irritations. Apply a small amount of organic coconut oil to the scraped or irritated skin. It soothes the area while protecting against infection and keeping the skin hydrated.

APPLE CIDER VINEGAR FOR MINOR INFECTIONS

Apple cider vinegar can be diluted and used to clean minor cuts or scrapes, helping to prevent infection. Mix equal parts apple cider vinegar and water, then gently dab it onto the wound with a clean cloth. Its antibacterial properties help cleanse the area while promoting faster healing.

Herbal Cooling Sprays for Hot Weather and Inflammation

Hot weather can be hard on dogs, especially those with thick fur or health issues. Herbal cooling sprays offer a natural and refreshing way to help your dog stay comfortable and prevent overheating. These sprays, made from soothing ingredients like peppermint, aloe vera, and cucumber, can provide instant relief from the heat and reduce inflammation. In this section, we'll explore easy-to-make herbal cooling sprays that will keep your dog cool, calm, and happy during hot days.

PEPPERMINT AND CHAMOMILE COOLING SPRAY

Peppermint is known for its cooling properties, and when combined with chamomile, it makes an excellent spray for hot days. To make the spray, steep chamomile in hot water and let it cool. Add a few drops of peppermint essential oil and pour the mixture into a spray bottle. Spritz your dog lightly, especially around their neck and belly, to keep them cool and comfortable.

ALOE AND LAVENDER FOR SUNBURN RELIEF

If your dog spends too much time in the sun, their skin can become red and irritated. A mixture of aloe vera gel and lavender oil can soothe sunburns and reduce inflammation. Apply this gel to your dog's nose, ears, or any exposed skin that looks red after sun exposure.

CUCUMBER AND ALOE VERA COOLING MIST

Cucumber is naturally hydrating and cooling, making it perfect for a summer spray. Blend fresh cucumber with aloe vera gel and strain the mixture to remove any pulp. Pour the liquid into a spray bottle and refrigerate for a cooling mist. Spritz your dog lightly, focusing on their paws, belly, and neck to cool them down quickly.

GREEN TEA AND MINT COOLING SPRAY

Green tea has anti-inflammatory properties, while mint adds an extra cooling effect. Brew a strong cup of green tea, let it cool completely, and add a few drops of peppermint essential oil. Pour it into a spray bottle and spritz your dog on hot days, especially after walks or playtime. This spray also helps reduce skin irritation from heat.

WITCH HAZEL AND EUCALYPTUS COOLING SPRAY

Witch hazel is a natural astringent that soothes irritated skin, while eucalyptus has a cooling effect. Combine equal parts witch hazel and distilled water, and add a few drops of eucalyptus essential oil. Spray it on your dog's fur to keep them cool and reduce any inflammation from heat exposure.

MAKING HERBAL TREATS AND CHEWS

Herbal remedies aren't just for first aid—they can also be incorporated into delicious, homemade dog treats for added health benefits. By making herbal treats and chews at home, you can support your dog's well-being with natural ingredients like chamomile, mint, and turmeric. These easy-to-make recipes combine flavors dogs love with herbs that provide calming, anti-inflammatory, and immune-boosting properties. Whether you're addressing anxiety or promoting overall health, herbal-infused treats offer a fun and nutritious way to care for your dog.

Easy Recipes for Nutrient-Rich, Herbal-Infused Dog Treats

Incorporating herbs into your dog's treats is a simple and effective way to boost their health with natural ingredients. These herbal-infused recipes not only offer delicious flavors but also provide benefits such as calming effects, anti-inflammatory properties, fresh breath, and immune support. From chamomile calming treats to mint and parsley fresh breath biscuits, these nutrient-rich recipes are easy to make at home. Your dog will love them, and you'll feel good knowing they're packed with health-boosting ingredients.

Chamomile e Oat Calming Treats

These treats are perfect for helping your dog relax and unwind. Chamomile provides a calming effect, while oats add fiber and nutrients.

Ingredients:

- 1 cup rolled oats
- 1/4 cup chamomile tea (cooled)
- 1/4 cup unsweetened applesauce
- 1 egg

Instructions:

- Preheat the oven to 350°F (175°C).
- Blend the oats into a flour-like consistency.
- In a bowl, mix the oat flour, chamomile tea, applesauce, and egg until a dough forms.
- Roll the dough into small balls or flatten it into shapes.
- Place on a baking sheet and bake for 20 minutes or until firm and golden.

Tips for Storage:

- Store in an airtight container at room temperature for up to 1 week or refrigerate for up to 2 weeks.

Turmeric e Coconut Oil Anti-Inflammatory Treats

Turmeric is known for its anti-inflammatory properties, while coconut oil adds healthy fats, making these treats beneficial for joint health.

Ingredients:

- 1/2 cup coconut flour
- 1/4 cup coconut oil (melted)
- 1 teaspoon ground turmeric
- 1 egg

Instructions:

- Preheat the oven to 325°F (160°C).
- In a bowl, combine the coconut flour, turmeric, and egg.
- Slowly add melted coconut oil and mix until a dough forms.
- Roll the dough into small balls or flatten it into shapes.
- Place on a baking sheet and bake for 15-18 minutes or until firm.

Tips for Storage:

- Store in an airtight container in the fridge for up to 2 weeks.

Mint e Parsley Fresh Breath Biscuits

These biscuits are infused with mint and parsley, which are natural breath fresheners, while the added nutrients support overall health.

Ingredients:

- 1 cup whole wheat flour
- 1/4 cup fresh parsley (chopped)
- 1/4 cup fresh mint (chopped)
- 1/4 cup unsweetened applesauce
- 1 egg

Instructions:

- Preheat the oven to 350°F (175°C).
- In a bowl, mix the flour, parsley, mint, applesauce, and egg until a dough forms.
- Roll the dough out and cut into shapes.
- Place on a baking sheet and bake for 20 minutes or until crisp.

Tips for Storage:

Store in an airtight container at room temperature for up to 1 week or refrigerate for up to 2 weeks.

Rosemary e Sweet Potato Immune Boosting Treats

Rosemary is rich in antioxidants, while sweet potatoes add fiber and vitamins to these nutrient-packed dog treats.

Ingredients:

- 1/2 cup mashed sweet potato (cooked and cooled)
- 1/4 teaspoon dried rosemary
- 1/4 cup oat flour
- 1 egg

Instructions:

- Preheat the oven to 350°F (175°C).
- In a bowl, combine the sweet potato, rosemary, oat flour, and egg.
- Roll the dough into small balls or flatten it into shapes.
- Place on a baking sheet and bake for 25 minutes or until firm.

Tips for Storage:

Store in the fridge for up to 1 week or freeze for longer storage.

Lavender & Peanut Butter Relaxation Treats

Lavender provides a calming effect, while peanut butter adds protein and healthy fats to these delicious and relaxing treats.

Ingredients:
- 1/2 cup whole wheat flour
- 1/4 cup peanut butter (unsweetened)
- 1/2 teaspoon dried lavender flowers
- 1 egg

Instructions:
- Preheat the oven to 350°F (175°C).
- In a bowl, mix the flour, peanut butter, lavender, and egg until a dough forms.
- Roll the dough into small balls or flatten it into shapes.
- Place on a baking sheet and bake for 15-20 minutes or until firm.

Tips for Storage:

Store in an airtight container at room temperature for up to 1 week or refrigerate for up to 2 weeks.

These herbal-infused dog treats are not only delicious but also provide various health benefits for your furry friend. Make sure to consult your vet if your dog has specific dietary needs.

Crafting Calming Chews for Anxious Pets

Herbal calming chews are a wonderful way to naturally ease your dog's anxiety. Whether triggered by loud noises, separation, or new environments, these treats combine soothing herbs like chamomile, lavender, and valerian root with delicious ingredients dogs love. In this section, you'll learn how to make these easy, nutrient-rich chews, offering your pet a natural solution to stress. Each recipe is designed to be safe, effective, and tasty, ensuring your dog stays calm and happy.

Chamomile & Peanut Butter Calming Chews

Chamomile is known for its calming properties, and peanut butter adds a delicious flavor that dogs love, making these chews perfect for reducing anxiety.

Ingredients:
- 1 cup oat flour
- 1/4 cup peanut butter (unsweetened)
- 1/4 cup chamomile tea (cooled)
- 1 egg

Instructions:
- Preheat the oven to 350°F (175°C).
- In a bowl, mix oat flour, peanut butter, chamomile tea, and egg until a dough forms.
- Roll the dough into small bite-sized balls or flatten it into shapes.
- Place on a baking sheet and bake for 20 minutes or until firm.

Tips for Storage:

Store in an airtight container at room temperature for up to 1 week or refrigerate for up to 2 weeks.

Lavender & Honey Chews

Lavender is a natural relaxant, and honey adds sweetness, creating a tasty and soothing chew to help calm anxious dogs.

Ingredients:

- 1 cup whole wheat flour
- 1/2 teaspoon dried lavender flowers
- 1 tablespoon honey
- 1/4 cup water

Instructions:

- Preheat the oven to 325°F (160°C).
- In a bowl, mix flour, lavender flowers, honey, and water until a dough forms.
- Roll the dough into small shapes or balls.
- Place on a baking sheet and bake for 15-20 minutes or until firm.

Tips for Storage:

Store in an airtight container at room temperature for up to 1 week or refrigerate for up to 2 weeks.

Valerian Root & Oat Calming Chews

Valerian root is a well-known herb for reducing anxiety and promoting relaxation. Combined with oats, these chews are easy on the stomach and perfect for nervous dogs.

Ingredients:

- 1 cup oat flour
- 1/2 teaspoon valerian root powder
- 1/4 cup unsweetened applesauce
- 1 egg

Instructions:

- Preheat the oven to 350°F (175°C).
- In a bowl, combine oat flour, valerian root powder, applesauce, and egg until a dough forms.
- Roll the dough into small balls or flatten it into shapes.
- Place on a baking sheet and bake for 20 minutes or until firm.

Tips for Storage:

Store in an airtight container at room temperature for up to 1 week or refrigerate for up to 2 weeks.

Passionflower & Sweet Potato Chews

Passionflower is known for reducing anxiety, and sweet potato provides a nutrient-rich base for these calming chews.

Ingredients:

- 1/2 cup cooked and mashed sweet potato
- 1/4 teaspoon dried passionflower
- 1/2 cup oat flour
- 1 egg

Instructions:

- Preheat the oven to 350°F (175°C).
- In a bowl, mix mashed sweet potato, passionflower, oat flour, and egg until a dough forms.
- Shape the dough into small chews or balls.
- Place on a baking sheet and bake for 20-25 minutes or until firm.

Tips for Storage:

Store in the fridge for up to 1 week or freeze for longer storage.

Ginger e Chamomile Calming Chews

Ginger helps soothe the stomach, while chamomile works as a calming agent, making these chews ideal for anxious dogs with sensitive digestion.

Ingredients:
- 1/2 teaspoon ground ginger
- 1/4 cup brewed chamomile tea (cooled)
- 1 cup oat flour
- 1 tablespoon coconut oil (melted)

Instructions:
- Preheat the oven to 350°F (175°C).
- In a bowl, combine oat flour, ginger, chamomile tea, and coconut oil until a dough forms.
- Roll the dough into small bite-sized pieces.
- Place on a baking sheet and bake for 20 minutes or until firm.

Tips for Storage:
- Store in an airtight container in the fridge for up to 2 weeks or freeze for longer storage.
- These calming chews are great for naturally reducing anxiety in dogs while providing them with a tasty treat. Always consult your vet before introducing new herbs to your dog's diet.

THE BOTTOM LINE

As you wrap up this chapter, you've taken some big steps into the world of DIY herbal projects for your dog. You've learned how to create your own herbal first-aid kit, so you're prepared for those little emergencies that can happen anytime. By knowing which herbs are essential and how to prepare them in advance, you can handle minor cuts and scrapes with confidence.

You've also explored simple home remedies for common issues. Whether it's providing relief during hot weather or making an herbal shampoo for skin irritations, you now have practical solutions at your fingertips. Each project offers real benefits to your dog's health and is easy to put into action.

And let's not forget the fun of making herbal treats and chews. Crafting these goodies allows you to use herbs in a rewarding way while strengthening the bond with your pet. It's a creative endeavor that both you and your dog can enjoy.

Now it's time to get hands-on. Try out these projects and see the positive impact they have on your dog's well-being. Remember to always prioritize safety and proper dosing. With a little effort and creativity, you can enhance your dog's health and happiness using the power of herbs.

Conclusion

As we reach the end of this journey through The Herbal and Natural Remedies for Dog Bible, it's time to reflect on the key ideas that have shaped this guide. From the very beginning, we set out to explore how natural remedies—particularly herbs—can play a vital role in improving the health and well-being of your dog. We delved into the science behind these remedies, the ancient traditions that support their use, and the modern research that continues to validate their efficacy. Through every chapter, our primary goal has been to empower you with the knowledge and tools to make informed decisions about your dog's care.

We began with a simple but important question: why should you consider natural remedies for your dog? Throughout the book, the answer became clear. Natural remedies offer a gentle, effective, and holistic approach to healing. They work with your dog's body rather than against it, helping to promote balance and well-being without the harsh side effects that often accompany pharmaceuticals.

We covered the many benefits of using herbs in your dog's daily care, from soothing anxiety and digestive issues to managing chronic pain and supporting the immune system. Each herb we discussed offers its own unique properties, and we explored how these herbs can be used safely and effectively to address common canine health problems.

The chapters on herbal medicine for dogs taught you how to incorporate herbs into your pet's daily routine, whether through teas, tinctures, or topical treatments. We showed you how to prepare these remedies at home, offering step-by-step guides that made the process simple and accessible. The goal was to help you feel confident in using natural remedies, no matter your level of experience.

We also examined the importance of working with your veterinarian and integrating holistic care with conventional treatments. By combining both approaches, you can create a comprehensive health plan for your dog that takes into account their physical, emotional, and mental well-being.

Finally, we explored real-life examples of how herbal remedies can be used to treat specific ailments. From itchy skin and digestive upsets to arthritis and anxiety, herbs offer solutions that are both practical and effective. And with the herbal encyclopedia and recipe sections, you now have a wealth of information at your fingertips, allowing you to tailor remedies to your dog's individual needs.

The motivation behind writing this book was simple: to offer dog owners like you a resource that demystifies the world of herbal medicine and shows how it can be used to improve your dog's health. In a world where pharmaceuticals often take center stage, it's easy to forget that nature provides us with powerful healing tools. Herbs have been used for centuries to treat a wide range of ailments, and they offer a natural, non-invasive way to support your dog's health.

I wanted to give you the knowledge to take control of your pet's health in a proactive, informed way. Whether your goal is to prevent illness, manage a chronic condition, or simply enhance your dog's overall well-being, this book has provided you with the information and tools to do so.

Looking back to the introduction, we started by discussing the growing trend of natural remedies in canine care. This trend is more than a passing phase—it's part of a larger movement toward holistic, sustainable living. As pet owners become more informed, they are seeking alternatives to conventional treatments that may come with unwanted side effects. This book is a response to that growing demand for natural, effective solutions that work in harmony with the body's own healing processes.

Throughout this journey, we have explored how herbs can be used to treat a wide variety of conditions. But more importantly, we've learned how to think about our dog's health in a holistic way. Rather than treating symptoms in isolation, we've looked at the bigger picture, considering how diet, lifestyle, and emotional well-being all play a role in overall health. By integrating natural remedies into your dog's daily care, you are taking a proactive approach to their well-being—one that is gentle, sustainable, and empowering.

Now that you have this knowledge, I encourage you to think about how you can continue to deepen your understanding of natural remedies. How can you apply what you've learned in this book to other areas of your pet's life? Are there opportunities to further explore holistic care, whether through nutrition, alternative therapies, or even your own lifestyle choices? The world of natural remedies is vast, and there is always more to learn. You might even be inspired to grow your own herb garden or experiment with creating custom blends tailored to your dog's specific needs.

Consider the role of prevention in your dog's health. Herbs aren't just for treating illnesses; they can be a powerful tool for maintaining wellness and preventing disease. How can you incorporate herbs into your dog's daily routine to support their long-term health? Whether it's adding a little turmeric to their food for joint support or using chamomile to calm anxiety, there are countless ways to use herbs proactively.

Now that you've learned about the power of natural remedies, it's time to take action. Start small—maybe with a simple herbal tea or a topical salve for minor skin irritations. As you grow more confident, try integrating more herbs into your dog's care routine. The recipes and guides in this book are here to help you every step of the way.

If you haven't already, consider talking to your veterinarian about how you can combine herbal remedies with traditional treatments. Your vet can offer valuable insights into how herbs can complement your dog's existing care plan, ensuring that all treatments work in harmony for optimal health.

Finally, continue to educate yourself. The field of herbal medicine is always evolving, and new research is constantly emerging. Stay curious, stay informed, and never stop learning. Your dog's health is a journey, and you are now equipped with the tools to make it a healthier, happier one.

As we close this book, I want to leave you with a few final thoughts. Caring for your dog is one of the most rewarding responsibilities you can have. Your dog relies on you for love, support, and guidance. By exploring natural remedies, you've taken an important step in providing them with the best care possible.

Remember, the power of herbs lies not just in their ability to heal but in their ability to prevent. By using herbs to support your dog's overall health, you're not just treating illness—you're promoting wellness from the inside out. Whether your dog is young and energetic or in their golden years, herbs can offer support that is gentle, effective, and long-lasting.

Thank you for taking the time to read this book and for your commitment to your dog's health. Your willingness to explore new avenues of care speaks volumes about the love and dedication you have for your pet. I hope this book has empowered you, inspired you, and given you the confidence to take control of your dog's health in a natural, holistic way. Here's to a healthier, happier life for both you and your beloved companion.

Made in United States
North Haven, CT
10 November 2026

22088885R00057